David G. McDonald   James A. Hodgdon

The Psychological Effects of Aerobic Fitness Training

Research and Theory

Springer-Verlag
New York Berlin Heidelberg London
Paris Tokyo Hong Kong Barcelona

David G. McDonald
Department of Psychology
University of Missouri
Columbia, MO 65211
USA

James A. Hodgdon
Department of Applied Psychology
Naval Health Research Center
San Diego, CA 92138
USA

Library of Congress Cataloging-in-Publication Data
McDonald, David G. (David George)
  Psychological effects of aerobic fitness training : research and
theory / David G. McDonald, James A. Hodgdon.
    p. cm. -- (Recent research in psychology)
  Includes bibliographical references and index.
  ISBN 0-387-97603-5. -- ISBN 3-540-97603-5
  1. Aerobic exercises--Psychological aspects. I. Hodgdon, James
A. II. Title. III. Series.
  [DNLM: 1. Exercise. 2. Physical Fitness-psychology. QT 255
M478p]
RA781.15.M33 1991
613.7'1'019--dc20
DNLM/DLC   91-4820
for Library of Congress   CIP

Printed on acid-free paper.

Camrea-ready copy provided by the authors.
Printed and bound by BookCrafters, Inc., Ann Arbor, MI.
Printed in the United States of America.

9 8 7 6 5 4 3 2 1

ISBN 0-387-97603-5 Springer-Verlag New York Berlin Heidelberg
ISBN 3-540-97603-5 Springer-Verlag Berlin Heidelberg New York

PREFACE

This book has two purposes. First, it is a critical examination of the question of how best to do research on the psychological effects of aerobic fitness training, and, more to the point, why this research is important. Second, it is a quantitative review of the previous research, with consideration of its impact on theory.

In dealing with the first question, we have included (1) some necessary background material on the nature of aerobic fitness itself and (2) a summary of the basis for the strikingly high interest in aerobic fitness in recent times. We then cover the fundamental questions of experimental design, with many examples of the sources of error or "confounds" that can be found in the fitness literature, and we finish by giving a list of recommended features for a well-designed fitness study. Our purpose is to assist in the design of future studies, while simultaneously providing criteria for evaluating previous work.

In dealing with the second question, we use a quantitative review process, *meta-analysis*, which is an objective method for combining the results of independent studies. Therefore included are material on the nature of meta-analysis, historical background, and strengths and weaknesses. The primary weakness of previously published meta-analyses is that they may suffer from lack of repeatability, due to incomplete reporting of the coding procedures and other data summary steps. We have therefore included much of our data so that the interested reader may easily repeat all of our steps, and add any other *post hoc* analyses or future updates of interest.

Conducting an objective assessment of this research gave us an opportunity to attempt a more comprehensive consideration of its impact on theory, or, more precisely, a theoretical model representing the established findings and their interrelationships. Good theory, by definition, promotes additional work that advances our understanding of natural processes. We hope we have made a contribution toward this end.

There are a number of compelling reasons for writing this book. Not the least of these reasons is the fact that interest in the psychological effects of aerobic fitness training is at an all-time high. Consequently, much has been written on the subject, but with mixed results. Fact and fiction abound with almost equal credibility and longevity, making it difficult to determine the truly established facts or plan intelligently for future studies. Our primary goal therefore has been to determine what findings have been well established, and what "findings" have not. In other words, where are we now, and where should we go?

We are speaking to anyone interested in the question of psychological effects of aerobic fitness training, whether as a consumer or as a current or future investigator. Investigators could come from a large variety of fields, including health psychology, exercise/sport psychology, exercise physiology, any of the health professions, and the disciplines of education, physical education, and sport. This certainly includes graduate students in any of these areas, especially students about to embark on a thesis or dissertation study, plus accelerated undergraduates. Doubtless there are numerous others, and we welcome interested comments.

We are especially pleased as well to have this opportunity to acknowledge the support and encouragement provided by others. Among the number of administrators at the University of Missouri and the Naval Health Research Center who made supportive contributions were several who were foremost. The project could not have been accomplished had it not been for the support provided by Laverne C. Johnson, in concrete terms of budget, space, and personnel, and also for the high compliment of his consistent confidence in our efforts. Similarly, Russell Geen, Eric Gunderson, and Joseph LoPiccolo each provided material and moral support, for which we owe our thanks.

A number of colleagues made substantive contributions. Paul Naitoh and Ross Vickers made critical suggestions in the early stages that helped us avoid serious pitfalls. Harris Cooper, ever the prototype professional, made significant suggestions in the early, middle, and final stages. He and John Honan read early drafts of several of tne chapters, and as a result some of our early mistakes were corrected in time. It is a rare privilege to work with such colleagues.

Still others went out of their way to provide technical assistance that proved to be utterly essential. Ray Hilbert and Richard Booth (Naval Health Research Center computing services), and Greg Johnson (University of Missouri computing services) were far more than helpful. Together they proved that a 2,000-mile gap between collaborative research sites can indeed be virtually eliminated.

Any literature review project is necessarily dependent on the facilities of a research library and its staff. We are especially indebted to and sincerely pleased to acknowledge the world-class assistance of Mary Aldous and Betty Croft of the Walter L. Wilkins Biomedical Library, Naval Health Research Center. Our sincere expression of gratitude could never fully repay their enormous contribution.

Finally, and most importantly, Merete McDonald provided consistent support and encouragement for the project, beginning with the first rough index cards ("just a quick little project"), and continuing through to its completion. Sharing with her all the temporary setbacks and moments of accomplishment in this work has been a deep and abiding satisfaction, and the gratitude returned is equally sincere.

David G. McDonald
James A. Hodgdon

January, 1991

CONTENTS

ONE

INTRODUCTION

The purpose of this book is to review and evaluate the research on the psychological effects of aerobic fitness training. It is a book that would have been impossible to write only a few short years ago. Today, however, there is a significant number of highly provocative studies on this question in the literature, with more and more appearing almost daily.

To accomplish such an evaluative review in a manner that makes a legitimate contribution, however, we must first address the background questions and more recent developments that have combined to make this work worthwhile at this time. There are indeed a number of such critical background considerations that are especially relevant, and it is our intention to clarify these matters first, and *then* turn to the target literature after the context has been properly defined.

In order of presentation, these major questions are: What are the public health considerations, especially with regard to coronary heart disease, that have led to the relatively recent public espousal of the exercise hypothesis, that is, that physical fitness produces a measure of protection from coronary disease? Are there any additional motivating factors, beyond public health considerations, that have contributed to the emergence of the national fitness movement? What are these other motivating factors, and what do we mean by the term "physical fitness" (especially *aerobic* fitness), plus how is it achieved, and what are the *demonstrated* benefits? What are the primary considerations in designing and conducting a rigorous experimental test of the effects of fitness training, and what have been the most frequently encountered difficulties with experiments in this area? How does one go about finding the published research on this question, and how best should one evaluate it?

Only after these questions have been properly discussed would it be appropriate to begin consideration of the research itself, including such questions as what psychological effects have in fact been demonstrated? What effects have not been demonstrated? Why? And, what are the implications for future research, that is, what are the unanswered questions that should be addressed next? Lastly, but far from least, what does this research tell us about the effects of aerobic fitness training? What can we say about its effects on coronary heart disease? Are we yet in a position of being able to provide a set of recommendations to maximize the beneficial effects and minimize the risks of coronary disease?

Clearly these are goals of great potential significance for both the psychological and the physical health of society at large, which in turn explains the critical need to set the stage properly by way of including the proper background material at the outset. Very few research problems encompass such broad areas of public health and lifestyle, fundamental laws of human behavior, experimental design, analysis and interpretation of complex and subtle effects, and far-reaching potential implications on numerous public policy questions well into the foreseeable future.

Coronary Heart Disease in the Twentieth Century

Obviously, coronary heart disease has long been recognized as the leading cause of death in the United States since the beginning of the twentieth century. Levy and Moskowitz (1982) describe this epidemic correctly when they point out that coronary heart disease:

> was responsible for nearly 650,000 deaths in 1978, and more than 150,000 of these occurred in people less than 65 years old. Approximately one-third of the deaths from all persons between the ages of 35 and 64 years are due to coronary heart disease, and nearly 40 percent of all deaths in white males aged 55 years and over are caused by this disease. (p. 121)

That this is essentially a twentieth century phenomenon is also very well documented. For example, less than 20% of deaths in 1900 were due to all of the cardiovascular diseases (including heart disease and stroke) combined. In stark contrast, however, tuberculosis, influenza, and pneumonia accounted for *more* than 20% of all deaths in 1900 (Califano, 1979).   Indeed, infectious diseases in general were much more frequent causes of death prior to this century.   Fortunately, in many cases (e.g., cholera, polio, measles, and diphtheria) these diseases have been virtually eliminated as causes of death in the United States because of revolutionary advances in public health practices, innoculation programs, and the like.   As a result, there has been a corresponding increase in life expectancy of more than 50% since 1900.   Males have experienced an increased life expectancy from 46.3 years at birth in 1900 to 67.1 years in 1970, and females have increased from 48.3 to 74.8 years in the same period (Lunde, 1981).   By 1984, these figures had increased to 71.1 for males and 78.3 for females born in that year (Bowen, 1985, p. 40).

Given this greater life expectancy due to fewer infectious diseases, it is not surprising to find that twentieth century Americans have been placed at greater risk for death due to the so-called silent killers - atherosclerosis, hypertension, lung cancer, and other malignancies that give no warning or other reliable signs during a relatively long period of incubation.   This increased risk was almost certainly accelerated by the changing lifestyles of Americans after the turn of the century.   Prior to the industrial revolution about a hundred years ago, farmers and others with a relatively active physical lifestyle made up a clear majority of the population.   Although there were many more daily hardships at that time, such an active life still seems to have provided a measure of protection, albeit inadvertantly, from major cardiovascular disease.

With the introduction of the internal combustion engine and other labor-saving devices, more and more Americans moved from the farms to the larger cities and adopted increasingly sedentary lifestyles.   We rapidly adapted to the use of inventions of convenience, including automobiles. Consequently, Stamler (1973) was able (quite correctly) to state that the:

industrialized countries are indeed being ravaged by an epidemic of coronary disease especially among males. . . .   Data show continuing high rates in the United States, with no further rises recently, but no evidence yet of a decline, at least not through 1968, the most recent year for which complete national data are available. (p. 5)

Naturally, the economic consequences of such an epidemic are of major proportions. National health expenditures have increased at an alarming pace in the United States. Since 1940, total expenditures have increased from 4.0% of the gross national product in 1940, to 7.6% in 1970, 9.4% in 1980, and 10.6% in 1984 (Bowen, 1985, p. 128). These percentages translate into $4.0, $75.0, $247.5, and $387.4 billions of dollars, respectively, for health expenditures for all causes. In 1984, this represented $1,580 for each man, woman, and child in the United States. For cardiovascular diseases alone, the estimated annual cost in 1981 was $60 billion annually, including both health expenditures and lost productivity. Clearly then, the use of the phrase "major epidemic" is in no way an exaggeration of the true magnitude of the problem created by coronary heart disease.

Can the Study of Risk Factors Reverse the Trend?

Matarazzo (1982, 1984) has raised the question of whether or not this society can afford to spend such a proportionately growing sum. A rather chilling observation can also be added at this point: Matarazzo (1982, p. 2) indicated that, by the 1990s, the projected health costs will be between 9.1% and 14% of the gross national product, although he thought the higher percentage was "unlikely." In fact, the observed cost in 1984 was 10.6% (Bowen, 1985, p. 128), and therefore the actual rate of increase is perfectly on track for the "unlikely" target of 14% in the 1990s.

Matarazzo (1982) argues persuasively that the reduction of this financial burden is a national responsibility shared collectively by all segments of society. Indeed, there is an alternative that can and quite possibly might still reverse this trend. Califano (1979) has graphically reported that, of the ten leading causes of death, "at least seven could be substantially reduced if persons at risk improved just five habits: diet, smoking, lack of exercise, alcohol abuse, and use of antihypertensive medication" (p. 14).

As is now widely known, the last two decades have witnessed intensive study into the role of "risk factors," that is, the study of the relationships between health and longevity and personal habits such as those described by Califano. Greatly expanded summaries of our progress in the study of risk factors have appeared in the annual reports of the U. S. Surgeon General, one of the more informative being that by Bowen (1985).

Encouragingly, some significant payoffs from the study and reduction of risk factors have appeared in national statistics on health trends, even though this preliminary good news has not as yet been followed by a downward shift in national health expenditures. More specifically, the good news is that, although the incidence of coronary heart disease showed a consistent increase in the twentieth century through the early 1960s in this country, the long period of increase was followed by a plateau in the middle 1960s, followed by a marked and highly significant decrease in the 1970s, that has continued throughout the 1980s. Such a turnaround is more than just encouraging. It might be one of the most significant developments in the history of the public health movement.

A number of articles, in addition to the annual reports of the United States Surgeon General, have been written about this relatively recent downtrend (Gillum, Folsom, & Blackburn, 1984; Levy & Moskowitz, 1982; Stamler, 1985; Thom & Kannel, 1981). All reports agree. As summarized by Stamler (1985, p. 11), age-adjusted mortality rates from coronary heart disease for all persons aged 35-74 rose by 14.1% during the years 1940 to 1967. However, from 1968 to 1981, the trend was reversed, that is, heart disease death rates decreased steadily, with the rate of decrease averaging approximately 3% a year over a reported period of 15 years -- or a total decrease of about 45%. Furthermore, the decrease was observed in all age-sex-color groups in the adult population, all regions of the country, and in both acute and chronic forms of heart disease. Although it is still too early to be certain of all of the factors contributing to the decrease, it is clearly evident that alterations in some health habits are major sources, for example, changes in eating patterns, decreased cigarette smoking, increased leisure time exercise, and behaviors leading to improved detection and treatment of hypertension (Stamler, 1985, pp. 16-18).

Emerging Significance of the Field of Exercise Physiology

It seems to be eminently clear and plausible, although not finally proven, that individual mastery over just a few health habits can have highly significant positive effects on one's likely risk of coronary disease.   Indeed, this message has undoubtedly been heard and heeded by millions of Americans in the last two decades.   Countless new products have appeared in the marketplace, on restaurant menus, in the newest cookbooks, and in feature articles in all of the media promoting all of the latest low-fat, low-calorie, and low-sodium dietary choices.   At the same time, newly passed local ordinances, public health programs, and the like, have all combined to make it more and more difficult to smoke cigarettes.   The varieties of exercise plans, programs, clinics, workshops, and similar opportunities are almost limitless.   It is now commonplace to see runners, cyclists, and walkers on the streets and country roads at all hours, in all seasons, and in all regions of the United States - something that would have been almost unthinkable only two short decades ago.   Although still a clear minority of the total population, the number of such exercisers has grown remarkably.

One of the greatest ironies of this phenomenon, however, is that it was *not* the study of risk factors, including regular exercise, that led to the national increase in jogging, running, and so on.   The risk factor studies have had great impact on such health habits as diet and smoking; however, the initial impetus for the widespread popularity of running came from an entirely different source.   What were the major causes?

First came exercise physiology.   Gillick (1984) makes a persuasive case for the notion that the field of exercise physiology emerged, not from the field of medicine, but rather from the intellectual roots provided by (1) the military, with its long-standing commitment to the concept of physical fitness, (2) competitive sports, especially with the increased experimentation in development of improved training techniques, and (3) work in cardiac rehabilitation, wherein it was recognized in the 1960s that repetitive, sustained exercise could be used as a means of improving the point of strain at which chest pain occurs in patients with angina.

Clearly the work in these diverse areas yielded significant payoffs, the results of which finally converged at a single point of focus, now recognized as the independent field of exercise physiology. The stage was thus set for the appearance of Cooper's (1968) book, *Aerobics*, which caught the collective imagination of the now ubiquitous exercising public. Although this volume was not by any means the first to recommend exercise to achieve fitness, including both physical and mental health, it was certainly the most successful at that time. The response was immediate. Not just the print media and the running magazines, but for example no less than the relatively conservative *Science* published an editorial in the same year (Abelson, 1968), recommending physical fitness as a means of making the heart more efficient and promoting an improvement in mental attitude.

Undoubtedly, another major contributing factor was the dramatic population increase associated with the maturing "baby boom generation," those born in the period from 1946 through the early 1960s, now often called "boomers." Without this large population increase, the trends and other changes that we have noted here would be hardly noticeable. As Jones (1980) has stated:

> When Americans went on a fitness kick, it was because the baby boomers were beginning to feel flabby. . . . Tennis boomed, but it was the jogging craze that brought out the generation in the greatest numbers. Millions of them were on the road. (p. 312)

Finally, Gillick (1984) argues that still one additional ingredient was vital, namely, the political disillusionment resulting from the racial unrest and the antiwar movement of the 1960s:

> The collapse of the liberal consensus -- the belief that the strength and virtue of America had created

peace abroad and harmony at home -- coming on top of a shattered faith that American medicine could render the world safe from disease, led to the view that America was morally sick, in need of spiritual renewal. (p. 375)

Thus the public was not only receptive to a new alternative, but it felt a strong need for it. Others, such as Fixx (1977, 1980) and Sheehan (1975), joined in, and the movement was literally off and running.

Can Fitness Provide Insurance Against Coronary Heart Disease?

Curiously, it was only later that the notion of heart attack insurance through running fitness received popular attention. Bassler and Scaff (1974, 1975) advocated marathon running for everyone, based on what is now recognized as the erroneous belief that such levels of fitness produced immunity from heart attack. Whereas this early belief was later shown to be untrue by Noakes, Opie, Rose, and Kleynhans (1979), it still left the exciting possibility that significant cardiovascular gains (if not fully preventive measures) remain within each individual's grasp.

Although slow in coming, relatively rigorous experiments, still in need of improvement, began to appear in the scientific literature. Reviews of the literature generally remained cautious in tone, recommending refinements in future research, but also offering the guarded conclusion that vigorous physical exercise is apparently associated with decreased risk of coronary heart disease.

Even though it is not the primary purpose of this book to evaluate the extensive body of published research on the question of the effects of exercise and fitness on risk of coronary disease, the reader is nevertheless directed to the most recent and comprehensive reviews of this literature. The conclusions reached at the end of each such review are most illuminating. For example, Eichner (1983) concluded that "the 'exercise hypothesis' is plausible, even likely, but still unproved" (p. 1008), whereas Haskell (1984) summarized that "men who select a physically active lifestyle on their own generally demonstrate fewer clinical

manifestations of coronary heart disease than their sedentary counterparts; when events do occur, they tend to be
less severe and to appear at an older age" (p. 413).   Haskell
also gives a detailed summary of the various physiological
mechanisms that have been proposed to explain the exercise
hypothesis, such as delay of atherosclerosis, increased vas-
cularization, decreased oxygen demand, and antidysrhythmic
effects.   Lastly, while also reviewing essentially the same
body of research, Siscovick, LaPorte, and Newman (1985)
concluded that:

> there is mounting evidence that habitual vigorous
> activity is associated with an overall reduced risk
> of coronary heart disease.   It is unlikely that this
> association merely reflects the "selection" that re-
> sults from sick persons who tend to be less active.
> (p. 180)

Thus, the reader may detect varying degrees of caution
and/or optimism in these concluding remarks;. however, it
would be incorrect to surmise that Eichner, Haskell, and
Siscovick et al. stand in strong disagreement.   Rather, it
is more correct to suggest that any apparent disagreement
is more likely to be only superficial.   In actual fact, each
of these reviewers is optimistic that the exercise hypothesis
will ultimately be verified without serious remaining doubt.
Toward this goal, Siscovick et al. include an important set
of suggested questions and recommendations for future research, including studies for specific dose-response effects
of exercise, effects on different age groups, longevity,
gender, and other risk factors, as well as studies on how
best to maximize benefits and minimize risks.   Studies of
such finely specified effects could, in the long run, provide
a great deal of needed substantiation.

Problems of rigorous experimental design and method
of subject selection also remain stubbornly unresolved.
Eichner provides a vivid description of the recurring problem of self-selection in studying the exercise hypothesis:
evaluations of existing groups always run the risk of simply
confirming the presence of prior extraneous selective factors.   In other words. a group may be superior in a given
characteristic simply because superior subjects chose to
become members of the group.   Those who enjoy physical

activities do so because they perform better in the first place and are more physically healthy, and therefore they are more likely to volunteer for an exercise study.   Subsequent events, such as level of physical activity, may or may not relate to any ultimate risk of coronary disease. Unfortunately, it is much easier to recognize this problem than it is to solve it, because an element of self-selection is virtually always present in studies of the effects of experimenter-induced exercise programs.   This is not only true at the outset of a study, as one seeks volunteers, but even more so later, after the usual subject attrition has occurred.   (See chapter 3 for a more detailed discussion of this problem.)

Exercise as Its Own Reward

All of the foregoing developments might seem to be enough to encourage the physical fitness movement, however, there is still another factor that has contributed significantly in recent years.   It was not until the latter part of the 1970s that the *addictive* properties of fitness emerged as an additional primary motivating force for the running movement.   Ironically, it was only at this point that exercise for its own sake appeared as an explanatory concept with significant frequency to explain the sustained behavior of runners (or any *endurance* athlete) -- far more than the numbers originally committed to the notion of running for insurance from heart disease.   Mounting evidence clearly showed that exercise was gaining in popularity, not only among middle-aged men at risk of coronary heart disease, but also among women and young people (Lambert, Netherton, Finison, Hyde, & Spaight, 1982).   For them, as well as for most other endurance athletes, running (or fitness) represented the best possible means of proving their profound commitment to the idea that the true route to individual health and redemption lay in "good, clean living" (Gillick, 1984).

Similarly, the notion that running per se could serve as a therapeutic vehicle for treatment of depression, anxiety, and other psychological ills (see Sacks & Sachs, 1981) was also gaining in popularity at a comparably rapid pace. Implicit in such a belief is the idea that, if running is a treatment for depression, it is also a means of prevention or, alternatively, of achieving the so-called "runner's high," a drug-free and effective method for reaching a new and greater sense of well-being never previously thought possible. Thus the greatest burgeoning literature on the effects of running is *not* in the area of prevention of heart disease, but rather in the psychological arena, as a treatment for depression, a safe means for a sense of well-being, and personal restoration and redemption (see Sachs & Buffone, 1984).

It was against this background that the decision was made to write this review addressed specifically to the question of the psychological effects of exercise, or, more specifically of aerobic fitness resulting from appropriate endurance training. Included in such a review must necessarily be a full consideration of questions of experimental design, measurement, and a final resulting view of established findings and remaining questions. Given the broad current interest and potential contribution toward physical and psychological health, it is hoped that this project will constitute a timely and helpful contribution.

Summary

The following events constitute the major factors that provide the background for the present work:

1. The national incidence of coronary heart disease, which maintained at consistently low levels up to and including the last century, increased to epidemic proportions after 1900 through the 1960s, due to increasingly sedentary lifestyles and the virtual elimination of death due to infectious diseases.
2. Mounting evidence has shown that reduction of so-called risk factors, such as diet, smoking, alcohol abuse, physical activity, and so on, can lead to drastically reduced incidence of death from coronary heart disease, hypertension, lung cancer, and the like.
3. The recognition that risk factors play a major role in the etiology of disease means that individuals can potentially assert substantial control over per-

sonal health habits as a significant means of prevention.

4. The advent of the field of exercise physiology,
    coupled with the political disillusionment of the
    1960s and the maturing baby boom generation, set
    the stage for the rapid public espousal of the ex-
    ercise hypothesis, namely, that physical fitness
    produces a measure of protection from coronary
    disease.

5. More recent research has shown that the exercise
    hypothesis is "plausible, even likely, but still un-
    proved," but there is mounting evidence that "ha-
    bitual vigorous activity is associated with an overall
    reduced risk of coronary heart disease."

6. The physical fitness movement, although originally
    introduced largely as an individual means of re-
    ducing the risk of coronary heart disease (while still
    assuming personal responsibility for one's own
    wellness), has come to be an end in itself, pursued
    because of the appeal of upright living as a means
    to personal and social redemption, as well as a
    therapeutic vehicle for treating depression and a
    host of other psychological ills, and a safe means
    of achieving a sense of well-being. Obviously, the
    personal and public health implications of such de-
    velopments are enormous.

TWO

AEROBIC FITNESS

This chapter is a review of the concept of aerobic fitness. How it is defined. How it differs from other kinds of fitness. What the difference is between aerobic and anaerobic fitness. What the best demonstrated methods are for producing aerobic fitness. How one establishes the validity of a fitness program, that is, prove that fitness was indeed achieved. And, foremost, after establishing that aerobic fitness has been achieved, what the most important beneficial effects are. Also, we consider whether there are differences between *claimed* benefits and *actually proven* benefits, and if there are, which of the many claimed benefits have in fact been demonstrated? In other words, are the returns worth the effort?

What Is Aerobic Fitness?

Aerobic means "in the presence of oxygen," in contrast to *anaerobic* which means "in the absence of oxygen." The essential source of energy in the human body is provided by the breakdown of glycogen (a carbohydrate stored primarily in muscle and in the liver) into glucose, a high-energy sugar. This breakdown of glycogen, termed glycolysis, can occur either aerobically (with oxygen) or anaerobically (without oxygen), which in turn *greatly* influences the resulting maximum capacity and power. Anaerobic glycolysis generally produces a relatively large amount of useful energy in a relatively short time followed very quickly by muscle fatigue and diminished capacity to continue the work or exercise. Any activity requiring rapid expenditure of large amounts of energy for a short burst generally relies on anaerobic glycolysis, such as weight lifting and short sprints (e.g., 100 meters).

Aerobic glycolysis, on the other hand, produces less useful energy per unit time, however, it does so over a much longer time. Consequently, the total amount of useful energy is actually about 75 times greater as a result of aerobic glycolysis than from anaerobic glycolysis. The presence of oxygen in aerobic glycolysis creates a condition of equilibrium or steady state, in which energy production and expenditure are in close alignment, which means that an individual can potentially continue a given activity for periods as long as several hours. Examples of aerobic activities could in fact include such sedentary activities as reading a book or watching a movie, since the steady state requirements of energy production and expenditure are met. Aerobic *fitness*, however, results from minimal training in such endurance activities as distance running, cycling, exercise walking, distance swimming, and the like.

In actual practice, most activities require *both* aerobic and anaerobic energy sources. Much of the detailed work on the biochemistry of energy production in living organisms lies beyond the scope and space limits of this work.

Popular Aspects of Fitness and the Exercise Revolution

Kenneth H. Cooper (1968, 1970, 1977, 1982, 1985, 1988; Cooper & Cooper, 1972) has clearly contributed far more than any other individual in popularizing the use of the term *aerobics*. He has defined this particular approach to fitness in somewhat different terms, although there is no apparent intention to distinguish this form of fitness from the definition of aerobic fitness discussed above.

For Cooper, the definition has varied somewhat, however, in general aerobics refers to (1) "a variety of exercises that stimulate heart and lung activity for a time period sufficiently long to produce beneficial changes in the body" (1970, p. 15), and (2) "those activities that require oxygen for prolonged periods and place such demands on the body that it is required to improve its capacity to handle oxygen" (1982, p. 13).

These beneficial changes or improvements are usually what is termed the *training effect*. Although the use of the term *fitness* at times seems to suggest an all-or-none state of physical conditioning (i.e., one is either fit or not), any degree of high, medium, or low fitness can (and does) occur, and therefore it refers to a continuum over which one can show progress, backsliding, or maintain a steady state.   Similarly, the training effect, depending on many individual variables, can be large, small, lost, acquired, maintained, and so on.   It is not correct to describe an individual as "trained" or not, but rather as "more" trained, "less" trained, and the like.

What Is the Training Effect and How Is It Achieved?

Much is known about the beneficial cardiopulmonary and musculoskeletal changes that occur as a result of exercise (the training effect), and comprehensive reviews have been written by Blomqvist and Saltin (1983), Clausen (1977), and Scheuer and Tipton (1977).   Guidelines published by the American College of Sports Medicine (ACSM, 1978) emphasize that the training effect is "complex" and includes many "peripheral, central, structural, and functional factors" (p. vii).   While positive changes in a large number of variables have been reported, lack of extensive in-depth data has caused the ACSM to limit the most useful training effect changes to improvements in VO_{2max} (maximum oxygen uptake), total body mass, fat weight, and lean body weight.

A rather large variety of possible exercises can be used to produce the training effect.   Many writers seem to refer to running as *the* exercise to produce aerobic fitness; however, any activity that (1) uses large muscle groups, (2) can be maintained continuously, and (3) is rhythmic in nature could qualify as an aerobic exercise.   This includes all of the following: walking-hiking, running-jogging, swimming, skating, cycling, rowing, cross-country skiing, rope skipping, handball-racquetball-squash, basketball, aerobic dancing, plus any one of a host of other possibilities that the imaginative exerciser could develop.

It must be remembered, however, that much depends on individual motivation, including not only the kind of exercise, but also the amount, frequency, and extent of exercise history.   Any one of the foregoing list of activities could be pursued in such a halfhearted or irregular manner that no training effect occurs, or, conversely, could be maintained sufficiently to produce excellent improvement in aerobic fitness.   One method of determining whether sufficient effort has been exerted is to monitor the increase in heart rate that occurs as a result of the exercise. In general, an increase of 60% to 90% of maximum heart rate reserve is necessary to achieve the training effect (ACSM, 1978). Much more information on how to calculate these predicted changes in heart rate is readily available in any current reference on aerobic fitness.

Virtually all of the available experimental evidence consistently shows that improvement in aerobic capacity is directly related to the frequency, intensity, and duration of training. The ACSM (1991) recommends that healthy adults exercise 3 to 5 days per week, at 60% to 70% of maximum heart rate reserve, for 15 to 60 minutes (depending on intensity). Fortunately, nonathletic adults can accomplish the same results with less risk by limiting their exercise to low or moderate intensity activity of longer duration. Training effects appear to be independent of the mode of activity, so long as the frequency, intensity, and duration of training are similar -- meaning that the total energy expenditures are similar. Therefore, any of the activities listed above may be potentially used to derive the same training effect.

What Are the Risks and Necessary Precautions?

Due caution is extremely important and should be maintained to avoid injuries and other problems, especially in the case of beginners, children, the elderly, and, most importantly, individuals with any of the symptoms of coronary disease, such as chest pain or hypertension, or any other physical handicap. For example, heat illnesses due to dehydration (e.g., hyperthermia, heat stroke, heat exhaustion, and muscle cramps) are not uncommon in distance running events. People who are most prone to heat illness include the obese, the unfit, those who are dehydrated, those unacclimated to the heat, those with a previous history of heat stroke, anyone who trains while ill, children, and the elderly.

Therefore, common sense and good judgment should be exercised, and individuals with questions or special problems of any pertinent nature should obtain a physical examination (especially those over age 35) and consult with a specialist in sports medicine. Beginners should be especially mindful of the fact that endurance exercise capacity should be developed gradually over a period of many weeks or months, with proper warm-up, cool down, and necessary equipment and clothing. Guidelines published by the American College of Sports Medicine on the nature of exercise for developing aerobic fitness (ACSM, 1978, 1991), as well as prevention of heat injury (ACSM, 1984) should be followed with care and good preparation.

What Are the Likely Results of a Fitness Program?

The foregoing section provides at least an initial background on how to begin an aerobic fitness program. But what is the likely target or end-product? In other words, what's all the excitement about?

According to the ACSM (1978, p. vii), training of sufficient quality and quantity can produce improvements of 5% to 25% in VO$_{2max}$ (depending on the initial level of fitness), plus a decrease in total body mass and fat weight, and no change or a slight increase in lean body weight. Interestingly, training programs with as little as 10 to 15 min of high-intensity exercise can produce significant increases in VO$_{2max}$, with no change in total body mass or fat weight, suggesting that one can have separate goals for oxygen capacity and body mass under controlled circumstances.

The real questions, however, are: What good does it do to increase oxygen capacity and reduce fat weight? So what? Was it really worth all that work? If so, why and how? It has been suggested in the preceding sections that there are indeed many other complex changes and improvements that accompany aerobic fitness. For example, Cooper (1982, p. 107) suggests the following:

1. Higher levels of energy for longer periods.
2. Improved digestion and control of constipation.
3. Realistic way to lose and control weight.
4. Bones that will continue to be strong with age.
5. Improved intellectual capacity and increased productivity.
6. Better and more effective sleep.

7.   A very effective way to control depression and other emotional disturbances.
8.   Relief from stress without the use of alcohol and drugs.
9.   Significant added protection from heart disease.

Notice that protection from heart disease is given last in a list of nine potential benefits, quite a shift from the earlier treatments (Cooper, 1968, 1970) where the emphasis was almost exclusively on the reduced risk of heart disease. Clearly, the change in motivating forces outlined by Gillick (1984; see chapter 1) is reflected in the more recent list. That is, personal wellness, including well being, increased energy levels, mental and physical health, and relief from stress, have become higher priority reasons for seeking and promoting aerobic fitness.

The contrast between Cooper's list of benefits and that endorsed by the ACSM is striking and certainly raises questions. How could two such different lists of benefits both be correct? The probable answer lies in part in the fact that the ACSM guidelines are based entirely on studies of effects demonstrated over the full range of frequency, intensity, and duration of training for proper use as comparative models. In other words, the ACSM guidelines are limited to only the most fully demonstrated effects of aerobic fitness training, changes in oxygen capacity and body mass, regardless of what additional effects may be observed under various special circumstances. On the other hand, Cooper (1982) understandably is attempting to list all more or less known effects of aerobic fitness training. The ACSM and Cooper should therefore be taken as presenting the minimum likely and the maximum known effects, respectively. If this is the case, then both sources are correct, but should be interpreted in light of individual situations.

Demonstrated Health Benefits of Aerobic Fitness

The primary purpose of this book is to review the research on the *psychological* effects of aerobic fitness training. However, we will skip for now that portion of Cooper's list referring to psychological changes, that is, improved intellectual capacity, control over depression, relief from stress -- almost half of the list. Similarly, the research showing how aerobic fitness provides a protective effect from coronary heart disease was reviewed in chapter 1. Excluding these topics still leaves a critical core of research on a number of potentially very important health benefits. Those that have been investigated most extensively and for which the findings are most clearly established include effects of aerobic fitness on the following:

1. Body fat and obesity, with implications for dietary habits and blood cholesterol.
2. Blood pressure/hypertension.
3. Blood sugar and carbohydrate metabolism.
4. Maintenance of bone density.
5. Quality and quantity of sleep.
6. Health habits.

The following is not a comprehensive review of all of the relevant studies of the health benefits of aerobic fitness training; however, every reasonable effort has been made to include the most conclusive reports, to demonstrate the basis for any given judgment that a particular health benefit does in fact occur. Research in this area is continuing in an accelerated manner, and therefore the likelihood of significant additional findings in future years is extremely high. Nevertheless, the following presentation is certainly intended to be representative of current knowledge in the area.

1. Body Fat

Aside from changes in oxygen capacity, probably no area of benefit has been more thoroughly established than that of reduced body fat. Numerous studies (see ACSM, 1978; Franklin and Rubenfire, 1980) have shown that aerobic fitness leads to reduced total body mass and fat weight, with relatively constant or slightly increased lean body weight. It is well known that continuous exercise of more than 30 minutes duration and with increasing heart rate of 60% to 90% maximum heart rate reserve utilizes more fat than carbohydrate. Therefore, if training frequency is maintained at a level of 3 to 5 days per week, significant overall decreases in body fat usually occur in 2 to 6 months

-- and thereafter in more obese individuals. This is the basis for the long-slow-distance (LSD) concept of exercise as the first choice when the primary goal is a reduction in body fat.

Still missing are studies of the *long-term* effects on body fat. For example, little is known about the status of obese patients 1 to 5 years or more after aerobic fitness training. Results of research in other areas would suggest that aerobic fitness might produce only temporary weight loss in some patients, but more enduring changes in others. The general finding in follow-up studies after treatment for any of the so-called addictive behaviors is that the relapse rate may reach 70% after 1 year (Dishman, 1982). More information on this question could be highly valuable.

Similarly, more research is needed on the possible interaction between aerobic fitness training and dietary habits as an additional basis for the reduction in body fat. It seems highly plausible to assume that individuals who actively pursue a fitness program will also be more likely to alter their food choices by reducing intake of high fat and other weight gaining foods. Some of the loss of body fat would therefore come from dietary changes, rather than the exercise per se.

Lastly, it has been somewhat disappointing to learn that the effects of exercise on blood cholesterol (fat) levels are best described as "inconsistent" (Bonanno, 1977, p. 277). For example, Bonanno and Lies (1974) found no effect of exercise on cholesterol in a study with carefully controlled diet and no weight loss. Hartung, Foreyt, Mitchell, Vlasek, and Gotto (1980) found significantly different cholesterol levels in marathon runners, joggers, and inactive controls (in favor of the marathon runners), which led in part to Cantwell's observation (1985, p. 635) that at least the trend is in the right direction. Exercise has also been shown to lower triglyceride levels more consistently, although the importance of this effect on coronary risk factors may be negligible since triglyceride has not been implicated as a risk factor as has blood cholesterol level.

2. Blood Pressure

The effect of exercise on blood pressure has probably been debated more than any other health benefit. Both epidemiological and intervention studies in well-controlled groups with randomly selected controls have been lacking. The few earlier studies generally reported no effect of exercise on blood pressure (World Health Organization, 1983, pp. 26-27).

More recently, Paffenbarger, Wing, Hyde, and Jung (1983) reported that Harvard male alumni who did not engage in vigorous sports play were at 35% greater risk of hypertension than those who did at all ages (35-74 years), and independent of a background in collegiate sports as undergraduates. Although questions of possible selective effects still remain, it appears that, even after statistical adjustments are made for level of obesity, more active subjects still show lower blood pressure (Cooper, Pollock, Martin, White, Linnerud, & Jackson, 1976).

Again, more research is needed. For example, Paffenbarger et al. have shown that physical *activity* is related to reduced incidence of hypertension, but it should be remembered that this is not necessarily the same as aerobic fitness. Such measures were not taken.

3. Blood Sugar and Carbohydrate Metabolism

A large number of studies have shown consistently that exercise reduces the symptoms of hypoglycemia in diabetics by increasing the tissue responsiveness to insulin. Many diabetics therefore need to reduce their insulin dose prior to exercising. Glycogen stored in skeletal muscle is depleted during exercise and replaced thereafter by glucose from the blood. This process and others serve to reduce the need for insulin production, potentially reducing insulin deficiency with age and subsequent diabetes (Haskell, 1984). Obviously, there are wide variations in these processes from person to person, and those with any question or problem in this area, no matter how seemingly trivial, are strongly encouraged to consult with a specialist in sports medicine or their physician.

4. Maintenance of Bone Density

The loss of bone calcium (osteoporosis) as a part of the aging process, particularly in females, is well known. Several investigators have shown that the rate of bone mineral decrease in females over 35 years of age averages a rate of approximately 1% per year (Smith, Khairi, Norton,

& Johnston, 1976), with the greatest rate of decline between the ages of 45 and 70 years.

There are a number of hypotheses to account for the
decrease; the two leading suspected causes are inactivity
and decreased calcium intake (Smith, Reddan, & Smith,
1981). Consequently, physical activity and calcium dietary
supplements are the most frequently prescribed and re-
searched treatments.

Smith et al. (1981) studied the effects (in separate
groups) of both exercise and calcium supplements in bone
mineral content and width of the radius bone of the fore-
arm, and Aloia, Cohn, Ostuni, Cane, and Ellis (1978) studied
the effects of exercise on total body calcium and bone
mineral content. The female subjects in the Smith et al.
study averaged age 81 years and completed an exercise
program of 36 months; the females in the Aloia et al. study
averaged 53 years and exercised for 1 year. Subjects in
both studies who underwent the exercise program only
showed significant increases in bone mineral content and
total body calcium. Since these groups did not increase
their dietary calcium, it must be assumed that the improvements were not due to increased availability, but
rather to more effective utilization. The one group in the
Smith et al. study that received calcium supplements in
addition to the exercise showed no greater improvement.

A plausible interpretation of these findings is that
physical activity places a relatively mild stress on the bone
which in turn stimulates a calcium enhancing adaptive response. It should be noted that these effects occur as a
result of physical activity in general, which presumably in
this specific instance includes aerobic conditioning. However, there is no known improvement in bone density that
is unique to aerobic fitness training per se.

5. Quality and Quantity of Sleep

Dating as early as 1966, a number of investigators have
reported that physical exercise has a positive effect on
human sleep (Baekeland & Lasky, 1966; Bunnell, Bevier, &
Horvath, 1983; Griffin & Trinder, 1978; Walker, Floyd, Fein,
Cavness, Lualhati, & Feinberg, 1978; and Zloty, Burdick,
& Adamson, 1973). Baekeland and Lasky's original investigation was a study of the effects of fatigue on EEG sleep
stages 3 and 4, intended as a measure of the hypothesized

restorative properties of sleep stage 3-4.   Ten college
athletes did indeed demonstrate significantly more sleep
stage 3-4 after strenuous afternoon exercise as compared
to the no exercise condition.

However, as pointed out by Griffin and Trinder (1978),
several additional studies have failed to demonstrate this
effect of exercise (or fatigue) on sleep.   A review of both
the positive and negative studies prompted Griffin and
Trinder to hypothesize that the seemingly elusive effect
of exercise was actually only observed in studies using
physically fit subjects, whereas those reporting negative
results used relatively unfit or nonathletic subjects.   Indeed,
as hypothesized, in their study comparing fit and unfit
subjects, it was found that fit subjects had more EEG slow
wave sleep (SWS -- stages 3 and 4 combined) on control
nights, and this difference increased more so after exercise.
Similarly, Walker et al. (1978) found more EEG sleep stages
2 + 3 + 4 (also termed non-REM or NREM) in male distance
runners as compared to nonrunners.

Reminiscent of problems in other studies of the effects
of exercise, some questions of self-selection effects must
be raised.   For example, Paxton, Trinder, and Montgomery
(1983) did not find a change in SWS of athletes in fit versus
unfit conditions, whereas Paxton, Trinder, Shapiro, Adam,
Oswald, and Graf (1984) showed a relationship between body
composition and SWS, although not in the same manner in
both fit and unfit subjects.   As a result, Trinder, Paxton,
Montgomery, and Fraser (1985) hypothesized that the nature
of physical training could be a critical factor affecting
SWS, a hypothesis that was tested by comparing endurance
runners (aerobic), weightlifters (anaerobic), a group with
mixed (aerobic and anaerobic) fitness, and sedentary controls.   It was found that the aerobic group showed more
SWS and NREM sleep than the weightlifters, substantiating
the original hypothesis of specific training effects on sleep.

These data are indeed persuasive, although some possible
effects of subject self-selection cannot be ruled out.   For
example, there may be differences between endurance
runners and weightlifters on a number of personality dimensions, such as sociability, motivation, introversion-ex-
traversion, and so on, and that these differences could in
turn be related to differences in sleep patterns.   Further
long-term studies of randomly selected groups would clearly

be in order, especially since the original notion (that aerobic fitness enhances sleep) could potentially be a significant drug-free means of reaching this goal, which would
be no small accomplishment in twentieth century society.

6. Health Habits

Cantwell (1985) has suggested that vigorous physical
activity and cigarette smoking are incompatible.   Thus,
although some individuals pursuing aerobic fitness continue
to smoke, they constitute a clear minority, certainly less
than the percentage of the general population who smoke.
Presumably, this reflects a tendency to adopt a generally
healthier lifestyle as a part of an aerobic fitness program,
that is, such individuals are more likely to alter a large
number of dietary, alcohol intake, and smoking habits in
the direction of a healthier lifestyle.

Unfortunately, however, large-scale alteration in health
habits does not in fact seem to be the case.   Even though
very few participants in the Boston marathon are smokers
(Cantwell, 1985, p. 634), this association is less striking in
more average exercise groups.   In fact, Blair, Jacob, and
Powell (1985) reported that, although there is a negative
association between physical activity and smoking, the effect is weak.   Similarly, the association with alcohol intake
has varied inconsistently from study to study.   However,
there is at least some reasonable evidence to indicate that
exercise is positively associated with positive weight control and judicious caloric intake (Blair et al., 1985).

It seems clear that changes in health habits are really
changes in addictive behaviors.   Therefore, brief changes
during the initial "honeymoon" at the outset of a fitness
program are to be expected -- with (again) the usual relapse rates near 70% after the honeymoon is over a year
later.

Undoubtedly, many such changes in health habits are
actually adopted as part of a general motivation for self-
fulfillment, of which fitness is only one part.   Thus, the
change in health habits may accompany the fitness program, but not be caused by it.   Further studies of these
processes could be of great interest and potential social
impact.

Summary

Research on health benefits of aerobic fitness has established the following primary benefits to date:

1. Protection from or delay in onset of coronary heart disease (see chapter 1).
2. Increased oxygen capacity (ACSM, 1978).
3. Reduction in total body mass and fat weight.
4. Probable decrease in blood pressure.
5. Improved carbohydrate metabolism, with reduction or delay in problems with diabetes.
6. Improved bone density in female subjects, whether from aerobic or any regular exercise.
7. Improved stage 3-4 (EEG slow wave) sleep.
8. Some temporary changes in health habits, such as diet intake, but less clear long-term benefits.

In general, all of these areas of benefit research have major questions still to be answered. The most persistent and pervasive questions revolve around the knotty problem of subject self-selection. Obviously, long-term studies of randomly selected subjects, with the broadest possible array of measurements taken on a repeated basis, could be of great value.

Lastly, one additional benefit of aerobic fitness has been deliberately omitted from this chapter, namely, the entire question of the psychological effects of aerobic fitness -- far beyond the initial question of effects on lifestyle, and the like. There is nearly universal agreement that aerobic fitness training produces significant positive effects on mood, self-concept, and various measures of personality, including anxiety and depression. Indeed, considerations of this nature make up nearly half of Cooper's most recent list of health benefits (1982, p. 107), and probably represents the most important component in the entire notion of aerobic fitness as a means of achieving total well-being. This is not only an enormously significant and complex question, but also the major reason for this book. A review of research on psychological changes is therefore treated separately in several of the following chapters (see chapters 6 to 10). Quite possibly the ultimate contribution of the concept of aerobic fitness toward the solution of any of the ills of society will stand or fall with the success of efforts toward establishing these broad psychological effects.

THREE

EXPERIMENTAL DESIGN

The essential purpose of this chapter is to review the most important considerations in the design and execution of a study of the effects of aerobic fitness training, especially a study of the *psychological* effects. However, many of the points to be discussed below are broadly applicable to research on exercise in general. Throughout the review of this subject, it is always our intent to exert a constructive influence on the design of future studies in the area, as well as the interpretation of any previously reported work. This is much easier said than done, and we therefore wish to apologize in advance if our tone seems unduly critical or unsympathetic at times.

In reviewing the work from this point of view, we have chosen to focus on a relatively short list of the most important questions that should be considered in any critical evaluation of the previous work, and also in the design planning stages of any future work. In this chapter, we have concerned ourselves with the following: problems with either subject or experimenter biasing effects in aerobic fitness research; problems with definition of terms and/or lack of standardization of procedures; problems with control of extraneous variables by means of rigorous experimental design; and how best to design a study of the effects of aerobic fitness training.

Introduction

No review of the psychological effects of aerobic fitness training would be remotely complete without a systematic assessment of the specific problems in experimental methods and design that are unique to this area of inquiry. As is true in virtually all areas of research with human beings as subjects, the problems in many respects are of such enormity that no set of practical solutions has as yet been devised. However, the mere existence of any such set of problems, no matter how overwhelming, cannot ever serve as a rationalization for sloppy, so-called "quick and dirty," short cuts. One can sympathize with an investigator struggling with the knotty problems created by lack of standardization, or the inevitability of subject self-selection effects, but it is more difficult to do so in the case of a premature report, based on "easy" data collected on a one-time-only basis from a single preexisting group. Examples of the former are inevitable, given our current state of the art, but the time has come when we should be far less accepting of the latter.

On the other hand, in defense of workers in this field, research with human subjects is never easy. Armchair criticism, however, often is. Therefore, it would probably be prudent to retain some measure of understanding of the size of the problems with which many investigators must live every day in the trenches. One person's compromise is another person's salvation.

This is especially true of research with subjects from noncaptive groups, most often self-selected volunteers who may or may not differ in many perplexing ways from the target population at large. Captive groups (e.g., those in schools, hospitals, the military, or other institutions) present other, but equally unknown, sources of bias. In general, these problems may be termed *subject* biasing effects; however, it should be remembered that there are also equally troubling *experimenter* biasing effects. Such problems constitute the potential array of extraneous variables, which (ideally) must be either cancelled out or else held constant in all groups. However, there is at least one alternative.

As Campbell and Stanley (1966) have suggested, the proper solution to such problems is often to patch up design weaknesses by adding additional observations to rule out, more or less systematically, possible effects of extraneous variables or "confounds." In other words, one can ultimately reach a point where the original independent variable constitutes the most plausible explanation for any observed effects. This then constitutes a genuinely constructive approach to bring one's findings out of an otherwise debilitating morass, and therefore it represents an approach that we heartily endorse, both in principle and in spirit.   This point is so important that we shall return to it later in this chapter.

What Are Subject and Experimenter Biasing Effects?

A subject or experimenter biasing effect refers to any source of influence that can affect the behavior of subjects or experimenters, respectively, in such a manner that it alters the outcome of an experiment.   Examples of these biasing effects in the aerobic fitness literature are extremely common.   In this context, a biasing effect is synonymous with an extraneous variable or confound, that is, any uncontrolled variable that can mimic, cancel out, or otherwise influence the effect of the independent variable on the dependent variable.   As such, these are sources of error that make the independent variable less plausible as the basis for any observed effect on the dependent variable. One simply cannot draw conclusions with confidence.   The independent variable may or may not have been the major cause.

On the other hand, just because a given interpretation is less plausible because of unknown effects of extraneous variables, it does not follow that the alternative explanation (that the results were *solely* a reflection of the extraneous variable) is somehow more attractive.   As a general rule, this is without justification.   There can be a world of difference in the meaning communicated by the notions of "less plausible" and "more attractive."   Plausibility refers to the relative level of probability or confidence one can place on an interpretation of results, and it is precisely this characteristic of an experiment that one can alter by addition of further observations and/or missing control groups to increase the plausibility of that interpretation.   We emphasize this point because other reviewers of the fitness literature have at times seemed to suggest that in fact the extraneous variables seemed more potent and therefore more attractive.   Perhaps we could term this a "reviewer biasing effect."

Subject biasing effects
Without doubt, one of the most common subject biasing effects in this research is the problem created by subject

expectancy, that is, subjects behave in certain ways simply because they perceive that they are *expected* to behave in that manner.   The interested reader is referred to a simple study by Nelson and Furst (1972) in which it was shown in an arm wrestling contest that the *expected* winner actually won the contest more often than the contestant who was in fact the stronger.   In other words, expectancy was more potent than actual strength.

Double-blind studies are not possible in fitness research, and consequently subjects *know* they are participating in a study of the effects of fitness training.   This knowledge alone can cause them to alter responses on a questionnaire from pre- to posttest, and modify any number of health habits, such as diet, smoking, alcohol intake, sleep habits, and so on, especially on a short-term basis.   Worse, these effects vary from subject to subject, such that some will alter their habits as much as possible, whereas others will not do so at all.

Several partial solutions to these problems are discussed in some detail later in this chapter; however, the problem is of such magnitude that a brief statement may prove helpful here.   Several possible manipulations are worthy of consideration, for example, experimenters can deliberately create low- and high-expectancy groups through the use of such techniques as highly optimistic versus highly pessimistic instructions to subjects.   Similarly, the effect of taking the pretest can be eliminated entirely (or at least measured) by adding a comparison experimental group that is given only the posttest.

Comparisons between different kinds or levels of training could also be highly illuminating, such as comparing runners with weightlifters, both at lower versus higher levels of training, since such groups will not necessarily differ greatly in expectancy effects.   Lastly, interviews, in-house (i.e., nonstandardized) questionnaires, and various self-ratings often lack the subtlety and degree of standardization necessary for measuring training effects.   On the other hand, standardized questionnaires, especially those with built-in measures of test-taking attitude, can provide a relatively objective measure of subject characteristics on various relevant dimensions.

Experimenter biasing effects

Possibly, the most noticeable experimenter biasing effect in this literature is related to the fact that many investigators are personally convinced of the beneficial effects of aerobic fitness training.   One cannot help but wonder to what extent this may have been communicated to subjects.   This is the Pygmalion effect of the realm of aerobic fitness training, representing yet another example of the classic self-fulfilling prophecy, namely, the fact that we tend to act in countless small (perhaps unconscious or thoughtless) ways to bring to pass that which we already believe.   In other words, those who are most convinced of the positive effects of fitness training will be more likely to observe such effects, as well as the opposite in the case of those who do not believe.

The only general solution is to rely on objective measures obtained in a standardized manner that is relatively free of biasing effects.   Some investigators may also have the option of using blind judges in certain circumstances, although the possibilities for contamination are quite real. In the long run, it seems likely that those who maintain a convincingly neutral position will have the greatest impact.

Problems with Definition and Standardization of Procedure

As in most areas of social or behavioral science, the aerobic fitness research demonstrates frequent problems of usage, definition of terms, and standardization of procedure.   For example, Hammett (1967, p. 765) correctly raises some question over whether athletic prowess is equivalent to physical fitness, a question that one can understand being raised as far back as two decades ago, but certainly one answered in the negative at this time.   His question is actually more properly considered today as a part of the larger problem that investigators of the effects of aerobic fitness training have not consistently included both before- and after-measures of fitness.   Indeed, studies still continue to appear with no assessment of initial fitness level whatsoever.   Given the fact that there are now a reasonable number of generally accepted measures of aerobic fitness (described in more detail later in this chapter), there is truly no justification for failing to include such measures in current work.

Similarly, although it may seem obvious or unnecessary, it must be emphasized that physical exercise, aerobic fitness, and running are not synonymous terms, in spite of the fact that they do overlap. Obviously, aerobic fitness training is but one kind of physical activity or exercise (compared, for example, with such anaerobic exercises as weightlifting), and running is but one (albeit one of the more popular) means of achieving aerobic fitness. For example, most of the studies of the effects of exercise on hypertension have dealt with physical exercise in general, whether aerobic or not (see chapter 2), and nearly all of the studies of the effects on depression have actually been studies of the effects of running (see chapter 7). It is therefore somewhat misleading, if not flatly incorrect, to state that some of these effects are due to aerobic fitness training, either exclusively or in general.

Effects of Extraneous Variables on the Validity of Experiments

When we say that extraneous variables or confounds lower the plausibility of the conclusion that the independent variable was primarily responsible for any observed effects on the dependent variable, we are actually saying that the extraneous variable has raised questions about the validity of the experiment itself. Obviously, then, the investigator has every incentive to try to minimize the potential effects of any such extraneous variables on the validity of an experiment.

Fortunately, for the investigator who is in the planning stages of any research in this area, a number of constructive strategies and (at least) partial remedies have proven useful. Campbell and Stanley (1966; see also Campbell, 1969; and Stanley, 1973) have provided the most cited and perhaps the most thought-provoking treatments ever published on design problems in the behavioral sciences. This includes a thoroughgoing analysis of the primary extraneous variables that may jeopardize the validity or weaken the integrity of an otherwise sound experiment. It cannot be emphasized too strongly that each and every one of these extraneous variables can and has at times affected the validity (and hence the plausibility of observed results) of studies on the effects of aerobic fitness training. The following summary description of these extraneous variables (or any good substitute) should be required reading for all investigators in the area, partly because of the universal nature of the fundamental problems and partly because an attempt has been made herein to relate each problem to fitness research in particular.

Campbell and Stanley (1966; see also Campbell, 1969) divide their list of extraneous variables into (a) those that affect the degree to which one can conclude that the experimental treatment made a difference, termed *internal validity*, and (b) those that affect the generalizability of results to other groups, settings, and so on, termed *external validity*. Those in the first group follow.

Extraneous Variables Affecting Internal Validity

1. History

Any events that occur between the pre- and posttest, other than the experimental treatment, could lead to history effects as an extraneous variable. When experimental and control groups are drawn at random from the same population and the pre- and posttest measurements are made over a relatively short time, the effects of history may be negligible. However, most subjects (whether students, patients, or athletes) do not live in a protected vacuum. If the experimental group is composed of self-selected volunteers and measurements are made over an extended period of time, then the likelihood of history effects must be considered. The number of possible examples is essentially unlimited. Time of the year, the start of fall or spring season, may have special effects on interest in training in the experimental group. It is always possible that replication with additional groups may help, most especially if a one-time-only event is suspected of having had some special impact. Some situations might also require a staggered system of collecting subjects, rather than observing all members of a group at one time.

2. Maturation

Any processes that produce change as a function of time, such as aging or fatigue, could be described as maturation effects. Curiously, studies of the effects of fitness training almost never include reference to possible fatigue effects, in spite of the fact that such effects could easily interfere with measures of fitness. Similarly, any disease/disordered process, whether it be depressed mood or atherosclerosis, follows a maturational course that could counteract or augment parallel processes due to fitness training. Many depressed subjects get better in time without much help at all, and therefore the lack of a proper untreated control group could make any reported recovery rates look much better than they actually were.

3. Instability

Instability refers to any unreliability of measures, caused by subject fluctuations and inconsistencies in measurement techniques. Although most measures of aerobic fitness are at least acceptably reliable, there are still fluctuations due to such variables as the nature of the instructions, experimental context, sex, age, and experience level of experimenter, and subject interest and motivation, or even the common cold. Estimates of VO_{2max} based on a treadmill test and a bicycle ergometer test will correlate highly, but imperfectly. Similarly, some of the standardized tests discussed in subsequent chapters have not shown sufficient levels of test-retest reliability to warrant their use in fitness studies.

4. Testing

Having taken a test can affect the scores of a second test, a jeopardizing extraneous variable in fitness studies. Included in this category are direct effects of the pretest, such as practice effects, which could influence posttest scores.

In addition, since blind fitness studies are not possible, subjects generally know they are participating in a study of the effects of aerobic fitness training. Therefore, the mere fact that they are asked to complete, say, a mood questionnaire suggests that possible mood effects are at least hypothesized, and this in turn could affect responses given on the posttest.

One possible solution, strongly recommended for consideration, is to include an additional group that receives no pretest.   Any group differences in posttests after training would then be presumably due to the pretest per se.   In addition, the use of relatively subtle questionnaires, with items sampling a broad range of attitudes and behaviors, as well as test-taking attitude, should be less susceptible to testing effects.

5. Instrumentation

Inconsistencies in measuring instruments and/or observers fall into this category.   It is especially troublesome in research areas that have not as yet achieved full, routine standardization of procedures, such as some important aspects of fitness research.

Examples of this problem are commonplace.   For example, blood pressure measurements are frequently taken with a sphygmomanometer and pressures reported in millimeters of displaced mercury.   Differences as small as 5 mm in diastolic pressures are often reported, in spite of the fact that errors of this size are commonly made when reading the mercury level descending in the glass tube. In general, since reliabilities obtained in one laboratory will not necessarily hold true in other settings, investigators should include such information at least once in published form after standardizing their procedures.

6. Regression Artifacts and Spontaneous Remission

Changes in measurements whenever subjects are selected on the basis of extreme scores constitutes statistical regression.   A clinical artifact that may appear to be very similar, even identical, is spontaneous remission, which refers to the fact that certain clinical groups may show improvement simply as a function of the passage of time. In fitness research, this probably occurs most often in studies of the effects of training on depression.   For example, subjects selected solely on the basis of extreme scores on a mood scale measuring depression would be expected to show some decrease on the posttest for this reason alone.   Given the lack of perfect reliability of mood scales, those who initially scored extremely high could only average somewhat lower scores on posttest.

In general, the best solution is to select depressed subjects on some basis other than their extreme scores on a mood scale. The mood scale scores then potentially become measures of the dependent variable, and no longer a part of the independent variable -- even though still susceptible to history, maturation, and testing effects.

7. Selection

Selection refers to the effects of differential recruitment procedures for experimental and control groups and is extremely common in fitness research because both groups are usually comprised of self-selected volunteers. There is no escaping the fact that most individuals who volunteer for a fitness program differ in many ways from those who do not volunteer, and such volunteers are also likely to respond differently to the fitness training itself. Therefore, the use of volunteers in aerobic fitness studies often raises as many questions as are answered. One possible solution is to place some volunteers on a waiting list by a random process, thereby constituting a no treatment control opportunity through the waiting period. Other methods of aggressively recruiting volunteers may become increasingly feasible, as knowledge of aerobic fitness becomes more common, although this alternative should be pursued with due caution.

8. Experimental mortality

Different rates of subject loss often occur across experimental and control groups because of the strenuous nature of aerobic fitness training, with its emphasis on endurance. Clearly, subjects are more likely to drop out of fitness groups because of various injuries, aches and pains, loss of interest or motivation, and the like, with the result that only those who perform better survive to the end of the study. Probably no single control group can solve this problem, but rather it places a great responsibility on experimenters to provide a safe training program with constant sensitivity to and adjustments for the various subject responses to procedures.

9. Selection-Maturation Interaction

Selection biases that produce different rates of maturation in experimental versus control groups could produce interaction effects of this nature. At the risk of sounding repetitious, this problem is common in studies using self-selected volunteers. For example, differences in motivation alone, not to mention recent events of potential historical significance, could easily produce different rates of maturation that could mimic any increased fitness effects. This could include temporary changes in diet, smoking, alcohol intake, sleep habits, and so on, all of which would increase the effect of fitness training in this group alone. By and large, the only real solution is to assign subjects to experimental and control groups by a random process and build in procedures to monitor or hold constant any health-related behaviors.

Extraneous Variables Affecting External Validity

The extraneous variables or confounds that affect the generalizability of results are typically more difficult to control or hold constant. It is therefore all the more important that due concern be given to these extraneous effects, in hopes of minimizing their intrusion as much as possible. The variables in this group follow.

1. Interaction Effects of Testing

This refers to the effects of a pretest on a subject's sensitivity to the independent variable, thus making the results for any pretested group unrepresentative for those not so pretested. For example, it is reasonable to assume that subjects who complete a pretest consisting of a mood and diet questionnaire will be alerted or sensitized to such effects during the period of fitness training (usually lasting at least several months), which in turn could affect these measures on the subsequent posttest.

Use of more subtle pretest measures may be of some assistance, however, it may be necessary to add a group that receives only a posttest after fitness training. This solution is discussed in greater detail later in this chapter.

2. Interaction of Selection and Treatment

Subjects may be selected who do not respond to the experimental treatment in a representative manner. It is well documented that variables such a socioeconomic status, education, and gender are highly related to exercise activities (e.g., see Lambert et al., 1982), as well as risk of coronary heart disease (e.g., see Eichner, 1983). Regular exercisers are more likely to be males from better educated and higher socioeconomic backgrounds, and it follows that this group will then tend to be overrepresented in any study using voluntary exercise participants. Generalization of any findings to lower socioeconomic and less educated groups would at least be risky, if not indefensible. Investigators can probably minimize the effects of this variable by using appropriate sampling techniques from larger, more representative populations.

3. Reactive Effects of Experimental Arrangements

Unusual or attention-getting aspects of the experimental setting may produce effects unique to the experiment, including the ubiquitous Hawthorne effect (the effect caused by a subject's knowledge of being in a study), plus any additional effects of nonstandard procedures. In general, the best solution is to remain sensitive to the responses of subjects, follow standard procedures in a professional manner, and provide proper reassurance and encouragement where necessary in giving instructions, debriefing, and so on.

4. Multiple Treatment Interference

Multiple treatment interference refers to any cumulative effects of prior treatments in an experiment where multiple treatments are applied. While this extraneous variable has been classically related to sequential studies of drug effects, it could also apply uniquely to fitness studies, since the training is given in an extended series of individual sessions. Processes such as fatigue, habituation across sessions, and possible social interactions between subjects, could all influence the acquisition of fitness during the training period. As with other problems, the best solution to this problem is experimenter vigilance and sensitivity to the responses of subjects.

5. Irrelevant Responsiveness of Measures

All measures of dependent variables include some error. This includes all pre- and posttest measures used in fitness studies, as well as measures of fitness itself. Use of standardized procedures, including published or standardized tests, plus samples that are large enough and properly selected, will go far in minimizing the effect of this problem.

6. Irrelevant Replicability of Treatments

In fitness studies, errors in treatment procedures would include use of an inadequate fitness training procedure. For example, it is well known that weightlifting and other anaerobic exercises have little or no effect on aerobic fitness. Certainly there is no reason why any study of aerobic fitness in recent years should not follow the ACSM (1978) guidelines with reasonable care in the choice of aerobic fitness training procedures.

Requirements for a Study of Aerobic Fitness Effects

Given all of the foregoing considerations in fitness research, it ought to be possible to identify the minimum experimental requirements for any study of the effects of aerobic fitness training. Even though there will doubtless be other factors in various special circumstances, it seems reasonable to expect that any minimally valid and useful study of the effects of aerobic fitness training will include at least the following:

1.   Random group assignment
2.   Objective subject selection criteria
3.   Measure of initial fitness
4.   Fitness protocol based on ACSM guidelines
5.   Objective measure of dependent variables
6.   Proper statistical methods of analysis
7.   Follow-up observations

If we can specify the minimum necessary requirements, then we can also develop a system for judging the rigor of any single study, an important system for the review that follows in the later chapters of this book.

1. Random Group Assignment

Subjects in experimental and control groups should be assigned on a random basis, as contrasted with studies in which the experimental groups consist of self-selected vol-

unteers. This is a vital requirement that calls for a full
explanation. First, "random" means that subjects are assigned to groups by a chance process that guarantees equal
probability of being selected for either group. As Stanley
(1973, p. 93) states, "One cannot overstress the importance
of assigning the sampling units *at random* to all of the
treatments."

Second, it is hoped that more and more experiments
will be designed in such a manner that they qualify as
"true" experiments (Campbell and Stanley, 1966, p. 8),
however, there are potentially useful alternatives, termed
"quasi-experiments" (Campbell and Stanley, 1966, p. 36).
The latter may be more feasible in many real-world situations where random assignment to groups is simply not
possible, and therefore should be seriously considered.

"Quasi-" here means *almost* or *nearly* a true experiment,
but lacking control over some of the extraneous variables
described earlier in this chapter, including random assignment to groups. A quasi-experiment may be possible even
though the experimenter may lack the ability to randomize
exposures, as well as control over the "when" and "to
whom" of exposure, but still controls the "when" and "to
whom" of measurement.

Quasi-experiments may be the best available choices to
ascertain some effects of aerobic fitness training, and
therefore consideration of this approach is strongly encouraged. Remember that some extraneous variables cannot be ruled out on the basis of only one quasi-experiment;
however, the alternatives can be rendered less plausible
as a result of an accumulated series of related (but not
identical) studies.

2. Subject Selection Criteria

Subjects should be selected on the basis of objective
(reproducible) criteria. This is especially true in studying
effects of aerobic fitness training in hospitalized, handi-
capped, or similarly unique groups, such as depressed or
postmyocardial infarct patients. Subject records should
include information on age, race, sex, height, weight, personal and parental medical history, education, employment
and/or socioeconomic status, and smoking and drinking habits. Subjects in all groups should be screened for medical
risk (ACSM, 1978, 1991).

Wherever possible, group means and variances for all initial characteristics should be reported. Although the assignment to groups should be by random selection, it can still be verified at this point that there were no significant differences in known extraneous variables, such as age, weight, education, or health habits, unless they form a part of the specific independent variable under study. .

Selection of groups by matching these variables is neither necessary nor feasible in studies with a large number of potentially relevant extraneous variables. However, some variables (such as sex) will obviously need to be equated by the experimenter.

3. Initial Fitness Level

There must be an initial measure of aerobic fitness level, as well as a second fitness measure at the end of the aerobic fitness training. This does not to rule out an additional group that receives only the posttest, as a means of measuring the effects of the pretest, nor should one fail to recognize that, in some circumstances, more than the minimal fitness pre- and posttests may be highly valuable.

Fortunately, any one of a variety of standard fitness tests may be used. Described later in this chapter, the most frequent choices are the treadmill test, bike ergometer, and step test -- each with optional maximum or submaximum protocols -- as well as the relatively inexpensive 12-minute or 1.5 mile runs. Blair (1984) has even suggested that, since heart rate is lower in more fit subjects for any given submaximal work load, any standard exercise bout of at least 3 to 4 minutes can be used to measure aerobic fitness.

On the other hand, even though it is known that aerobic fitness is associated with reduced body fat and slower heart rate, such measures as skin folds and *resting* heart rate alone can not be used as measures of aerobic fitness. Changes in these measures could be produced by other processes, such as diet changes or habituation to the experimental procedures, although the data should still be reported if available.

4. Fitness Protocol

The aerobic fitness protocol, as an experimental treatment designed by the investigator, should follow ACSM guidelines for frequency, intensity, duration, and mode of exercise for at least 15 to 20 weeks (ACSM, 1978, 1991). That is, the exercise should consist of any of the recommended large muscle, rhythmic activities (walking, running, cycling, swimming, etc.) for 3 to 5 days per week, at 60% to 70% of maximum heart rate, for at least 15 to 60 minutes of continuous aerobic activity.

Special precautions should be taken if subjects are beginning exercisers, aged, patients with physical or medical handicaps, or those with any symptoms of coronary heart disease. Most studies of aerobic fitness effects, especially in recent years, either meet the ACSM requirements or else come extremely close with regard to frequency, intensity, and duration, as well as recommended precautions for special groups. However, very few reported studies go beyond the minimum of 15 to 20 weeks of training. Undoubtedly, there are many practical and unavoidable reasons why this is so, yet the result is that far less is known about the effects of an extended program of aerobic fitness training over a period of many months or longer. More information is clearly needed about the causes of subject attrition, novelty effects that might disappear after the early months, prevention of injuries, and so on, especially as related to groups that differ in age, sex, education, health, exercise experience, and so on.

5. Choice of Dependent Variables

It should be self-evident that the dependent variables must be objective and reproducible, at the very least. However, a cursory review of the published studies on the psychological effects of aerobic fitness training clearly indicates that this is not always the case. It is more than a little disconcerting to discover that some published studies, although clearly the product of considerable effort and expense, fail to make a contribution solely because of a poor choice of instrument to measure aerobic training effects.

Examples include any nonstandardized procedure that is not reproducible by other investigators, such as open-ended interviews, in-house self-rating questionnaires, or projective tests. This is not to say that interviews and questionnaires could not prove useful in assessing behaviors such as exercise habits (Blair, 1984). However, the lack of accessibility and problems with reliability or validity of these methods in assessing so-called psychological characteristics (including attitudes, mood states, character traits, etc.) is called into question.

Results from such techniques vary from one setting to another because of differences in administration, lack of objective scoring, and failure to control for or measure test-taking attitudes objectively. It is therefore recommended that only standardized tests be used to measure psychological effects of aerobic fitness training.

Such tests are usually published commercially and are available to qualified users with norms and objective instructions for administration and scoring, plus other accoutrements of standardization. They are also constructed by experienced workers with no vested interest in studying the effects of aerobic fitness training.

Naturally, there are exceptions to these typical advantages, and the field of psychological testing has its limitations. As any reader of the *Mental Measurements Yearbook* (any edition) will know, the standardization and established validity of many "standardized" tests is often disappointing. Most tests do not have built-in validity scales and many more are highly susceptible to subject response sets. This is especially troublesome in fitness research, because the purpose of many questionnaires can be highly transparent. There is also at least one important area of research wherein studies based on interviews were more significant than those based on a questionnaire (Contrada, Wright, & Glass, 1985)!

Nevertheless, such standardized tests still provide the most objective means of assessing the psychological effects of aerobic fitness training at this time.

6. *Methods of Analysis*

It is not the purpose of this work to review the proper use of statistical techniques in the analysis of the results of experiments. This is *not* to say, however, that there are no problems. Therefore, some emphasis is appropriate at this point to stress the importance of proper statistical methods. Campbell and Stanley (1966) discuss many of the appropriate methods with each of the experimental designs that they present, and Silva and Shultz (1984) discuss some of the specific problems of analysis that are unique to studies of the effects of running (pp. 313-314).   Since current statistical texts and qualified statistical consultants are both widely available, there is very little justification for any use of inappropriate statistical methods, regardless of the training and background of the investigator.

7. *Longitudinal Observations*

The point was made earlier in this chapter that observations of relatively long-term training effects (more than 20 weeks) are seldom made.   Granted that this is often expensive and time consuming, and may be totally unnecessary in some experiments, it still should be recognized that appropriate follow-up of, say, 6 to 12 months, represents one of the most frequently omitted opportunities in aerobic fitness research.   Most of our information is actually about effects within a relatively short time, often less than 4 to 5 months.   Therefore, although follow-up observations can not be stressed with the same sense of urgent concern as some of the other problems discussed above, consideration of this possibility is strongly encouraged.

Procedures for Measurement of Aerobic Fitness

The final topic of methodological concern in this chapter is how best to measure aerobic fitness. We have alluded to this question in previous sections of this book; however, it is clearly important enough to merit separate treatment here.

The most generally accepted measure of aerobic fitness is maximum oxygen uptake (VO_{2max}). In the case of laboratory assessment of VO_{2max}, subjects are required to perform work on an apparatus, called an ergometer, used for measuring the physiological effects of exercise. The most common ergometers are the treadmill, the stationary bicycle, and the step test (as on a staircase).

Subjects are instructed to perform successively higher work loads until they reach a point of exhaustion, at which point the oxygen uptake is at its greatest value, hence the label VO_{2max}. Measurement of VO_{2max} requires determination of oxygen and carbon dioxide exhaled. Calculation of oxygen uptake is relatively simple, since the composition of the atmosphere is known. It is also necessary to monitor EKG and heart rate at the same time, hence the total associated equipment is not exactly elementary.

Standard recommended protocols have been developed for the treadmill (both walking and running), the bike ergometer, and the step test (ACSM, 1991). The treadmill is the most favored procedure; however, it is also the most expensive and time consuming. In addition, maximum-effort tests in general are *not* recommended for subjects in various higher risk categories (ACSM, 1991, pp. 1-10), and the lack of qualified technical and medical personnel may further prohibit VO_{2max} testing in some laboratory settings. For these reasons, it is often preferable to substitute one of the submaximal exercises in order to reduce risks and costs of testing. Such submaximal tests require the measurement of heart rate under standard work load conditions short of the point of exhaustion required to measure VO_{2max}. Standard work load protocols and formulae have been developed for converting submaximal data to a predicted VO_{2max}, and the general accuracy of these predicted VO_{2max} values, although far from perfect for diagnostic purposes in individual cases, is still acceptable for pre- and postmeasures of group aerobic fitness (ACSM, 1991, pp. 39-43).

For field testing of aerobic fitness, there are two commonly used measures: the 12-minute run and the 1.5 mile run. The 12-minute run was initially developed by Cooper (see Cooper, 1968, 1982) in his early fitness research for the United States Air Force. The only requirement is a flat running surface, such as an oval track, over which to measure how far subjects can run in 12 minutes. Norms have been developed for different levels of fitness, as well as age and sex of the runners. Similarly, the 1.5 mile run has been widely adopted by the United States armed forces as an indicator of fitness. Both of these field test techniques have the advantage of simplicity in administration, making them practical in experiments with relatively large groups. Although there is some loss in accuracy, such field tests are certainly an acceptable means of assessing initial and final levels of aerobic fitness in appropriate groups.

Finally, Blair (1984) has suggested that, because heart rates obtained during submaximal work can be used to monitor changes in fitness, it follows that virtually any standard (i.e., consistent) exercise of at least 3 to 4 minutes can be used to measure changes in aerobic fitness, whether in a laboratory or in the field. In general, we would agree with this suggestion, so long as the usual precautions are followed, and the requirements for standardization are met. After all, it is vastly more important to show that subjects have improved their ability to "run around the block" than it is to show that it was a "standard" block.

However, while simple alternatives do have certain advantages, there are limits beyond which acceptable measures of aerobic fitness may not be possible. For example, it is known that aerobic fitness reduces fat weight and produces a lower resting heart rate. It does not follow, however, that such measures as skin folds for body fat or resting heart rate can be used to measure aerobic fitness. Reduced body fat could be the result of a concurrent change in dietary habits, and it has been shown to correlate only moderately with VO_{2max}.

In addition, resting heart rate is subject to the pervasive effects of habituation to the experimental setting, in addition to any effect of aerobic fitness, hence it too is not recommended for use as a criterion measure. This is not to say that skin-fold and resting-heart-rate data should be routinely omitted from published reports. Quite the contrary, but such measures should not be the sole basis for establishing that aerobic conditioning was accomplished in the training program.

Summary

It is strongly recommended that the following considerations be given high priority in planning or evaluating any research on the effects of aerobic fitness training:

1. There must be clear recognition of the potential role of both subject and experimenter biasing effects as extraneous variables or confounds.
2. The possible effect of extraneous variables on the internal and external validity should also be recognized. Where feasible, opportunities to conduct

quasi-experiments, in contrast to pseudo-experiments (which we refer to as "survey studies"), should be fully exploited. True experiments, generally the most difficult to accomplish, should still constitute the long range goal.

3. Wherever possible, studies of the effects of aerobic fitness training should include all (or nearly all) of the following minimum requirements:

    a. Random group assignment.
    b. Objective subject selection criteria.
    c. Pre- and postmeasures of fitness.
    d. Standard aerobic fitness training program.
    e. Objective dependent variables.
    f. Proper statistical methods.
    g. Long term follow-up observations.

4. Procedures for measuring aerobic fitness levels should follow recognized standard procedures, or, at the very least, consist of a valid assessment of aerobic fitness in a reproducible manner.

FOUR

META-ANALYSIS

As we have stated repeatedly, the purpose of this book is to review the research on the psychological effects of aerobic fitness training. For this purpose, we use a quantitative reviewing technique termed *meta-analysis*. This approach to literature reviews is relatively new, and the reader might be somewhat unfamiliar with the logic and method of meta-analysis. Therefore, before dealing with the review itself, it was deemed appropriate to acquaint the reader with the historical background, development, and methods unique to meta-analysis, with special emphasis on the differences between this approach and that of more traditional research reviews.

The most important questions to be dealt with in this chapter are: How does meta-analysis differ from traditional research review? How and when did this approach originate? What are the strengths and benefits of meta-analysis? When is it most appropriate? When not? Are there lingering unsolved problems? And, if so, how should one deal with them?

The Nature of Evidence in the Scientific Process

It is widely recognized that scientific evidence, especially in the social sciences, is most often available or communicated by two different methods: primary and secondary reports. Primary research reports, usually the results of single or several highly related experiments, represent the fundamental units or building blocks in the scientific enterprise. They are the articles that comprise nearly all of the contents of most scientific journals, and indeed it is for this reason that most journals were founded.

There is probably no way to overemphasize the importance of such primary reports. The most basic nature of progress in any scientific endeavor occurs as a result of the accumulated evidence from a series of primary reports.

and, conversely, progress simply would not occur without them.

Ironically, however, it is quite rare in the social sciences to see any single experiment serve in a truly pivotal or decisive role, most especially if it represents but one in a series of similar experiments. As Lykken (1968) has summarized:

> The finding of statistical significance [in a single experiment] is perhaps the least important attribute of a good experiment; it is *never* a sufficient condition for concluding that a theory has been corroborated, that a useful empirical fact has been established with reasonable confidence. . . . (p. 158)

In other words, the results of single experiments become important only as they are a part of an ongoing series of experiments. This implies some degree of independent replication, conceptual expansion, and/or theoretical refinement, hopefully with some variety of subjects and methods.

In addition, whenever a series of experiments on a related question has been published in the scientific literature, there exists some potential opportunity for the so-called secondary report -- the research review. Research reviews. by definition, are aggregations of primary reports for purposes of analysis of findings and synthesis (ideally) into some new whole or corpus representing the revised state of the art. As such, research reviews serve a purpose that is at least as important as that served by single experiments -- in spite of the opprobrium implicit in referring to such reviews as "secondary" reports.

A truly valuable research review should provide at least a critical integration and interpretation of the published research in a given area. Methodological problems in design or measurement, if they exist, should receive special attention, which in turn should at least imply the proper corrective steps. Similarly, it should be made clear which questions, with what degree of confidence, have been answered and which have not. And, finally, it should then be possible to make more informed decisions on future strategies, that is. what questions need further replication. what questions have been answered (and therefore deserve elaboration), and what questions might best be discarded or revised drastically? Surely little argument is necessary to convince the greatest skeptic of the importance of such contributions. Many thousands of such reviews have been published in the scientific literature, and there is certainly every reason to expect that this critical process will continue in the future.

Indeed, there are healthy signs that the role of the research review has been enhanced in recent years, a turn of events that is not only encouraging, but also overdue. The research review as traditionally conducted has not been without serious problems, and it now appears that important solutions to some of these problems have been introduced.

Sources of Error in Narrative Research Reviews

In spite of the importance of narrative research reviews, the process of reviewing has been a subjective one. Traditionally, reviews have generally been limited to *narrative* summaries of research, however brilliant and illuminating they may have been.

The subjective nature of the review process can and does take several forms. Reviewers are free to use any bias, whether explicit or implicit, in deciding which primary reports or individual experiments to include or exclude, by whatever criteria, and in judging which studies were rigorous and which studies were not. Inevitably, this process results in some loss of data and an imprecise weighting of results at best, or the risk of misleading and incorrect conclusions at worst.

Several writers have shown that narrative reviews are consistently vulnerable to a systematic tendency to *under*estimate the degree of reported support for a hypothesis in the literature. That is, traditional reviewers are more likely to conclude that there is no (or only weak) support for a hypothesis, when in fact the degree of reported support is much stronger.

There are several contributing reasons for this error. As Light and Smith (1971) point out, narrative reviewers have often used the "vote counting" or "box score" method of combining the results of a number of studies, a method with several inherent problems. Such a box score method usually consists of a more or less numerical count of the number of studies reporting each possible outcome, with the "winner" being determined by the most frequent result. This method is implicitly based on the fallacious assumption that a "real" effect will tend to be demonstrated in nearly all experimental tests, or, conversely, a treatment that has no effect on a given measure will yield negative (or chance) results in all experimental tests.   That is, an all-or-none dichotomy is assumed.   This assumption is indefensible if the treatment effect is real, but still not overwhelming, as is often the case in social science research.

For example, Cooper and Rosenthal (1980) have shown convincingly that reviewers using *statistical* methods can in fact perceive more support in the literature and estimate a larger magnitude of effects than narrative reviewers working from the same primary reports.   Furthermore, Hedges and Olkin (1985, pp. 2-14, 48-52) have provided a thorough analysis of the fallacious nature of vote-counting methods.   Instead of an all-or-none dichotomy, it can be shown that the number of studies reporting significant results should approach the power of the statistical test as the number of studies becomes large.   *Power* is defined as the probability of correctly rejecting the null hypothesis for any possible true difference.   Thus, with sample sizes less than 50, and only modest treatment effects, the proportion of studies reporting significant results will nearly always be less than 50%!

Other problems with the box score method also exist. A simple count of significance tests ignores the effect of sample size, clearly a factor that could lead to rejection of the null hypothesis in one study with a large sample, and the opposite in another study with a small sample. Similarly, studies reporting large magnitude of effect should receive more emphasis than that provided by a simple count.   And finally, much information can be lost if the count aggregates studies that used different measures as the dependent variables, plus additional independent variables of potential interest (e.g., age, gender, education, socioeconomic status, etc.) in a single enumeration or box score.   The inherent riskiness of box score methods of literature review therefore seems eminently clear.

Origin of and Early Work in Meta-analysis

It is precisely for these reasons that the technique known as meta-analysis was introduced as an objective alternative method of literature review. Although it has not gone unchallenged (e.g., see Eysenck, 1978; Jackson, 1980; Mansfield & Busse, 1977; Marshall, 1980), the technique has gained widespread acceptance and has developed rapidly. The term *meta-analysis* was first used by Glass (1976) to refer to the principle of applying conventional statistical techniques to summarize the findings of a number of studies on a similar problem. The intent was to use quantitative methods to avoid the fallacies of the vote-counting method, plus other difficulties arising from the inherently subjective nature of traditional and other narrative reviews. Meta-analysis is an "analysis of analyses," a transcending examination of a scientific complex, its elements, and their relationships. Curiously, it is ideally as much a synthesis, as well as an analysis, of existing data, even though the name fails to make this clear.

However modest Glass' original intent in the use of the term, the label meta-analysis has stuck. Indeed, it has caught the attention of many writers with unusual speed and enthusiasm (Glass, McGaw, & Smith, 1981; pp. 24-56). Of course, this is *not* to say that there were no antecedents. For a more detailed description of some of these background features, the interested reader is referred to Bangert-Drowns (1986), Cooper (1989), Green and Hall (1984), Fiske (1983), and Wortman (1983), to name only a few sources.

Not surprisingly, there has been a dramatic surge in the literature on meta-analysis in recent years. Technical problems and questions raised by early critics have generally been addressed one by one, providing an excellent example of the birth, early growing pains, and first signs of maturing of a new technique in social research methodology. All of this began, however, with the first meta-analysis published by Smith and Glass (1977). They showed that psychotherapy is *generally* effective, disregarding the specific type or school of therapy employed. Such a report would obviously receive much attention for this reason alone.

However, the methods applied by Smith and Glass in summarizing nearly 400 studies of psychotherapy outcome were equally important in this case. Studies were coded on a number of therapist, client, outcome, and quality-related characteristics for comparison as independent variables in the meta-analysis. The results, or dependent variables, were converted into the *effect size*, that is, the mean difference between the treated and control subjects divided by the standard deviation. In this manner, the magnitude of the treatment effect was converted into standard deviation units, an approach with many advantages discussed more fully below. Suffice it to say at this point, however, that the approach of meta-analysis provided a new application of existing statistical tools in a manner that produced new and important insights from existing data. Smith and Glass (1977) summarize this point quite well:

> Scholars and clinicians [have been] in the rather embarrassing position of knowing less than has been proven, because knowledge, atomized and sprayed across a vast landscape of journals, books, and reports, has not been accessible. (p. 760)

Strengths and Benefits of Meta-analysis

Given that meta-analysis has provoked a great deal of interest, debate, and methodological revision and refinement in the literature (not to mention a host of meta-analyses), it is obvious that there must be a clear set of advantages to this approach. Indeed, such is the case. The following discussion will almost inevitably omit some beneficial details of meta-analysis; however, it is our considered opinion that the most important strengths and benefits of meta-analysis are as follows:

1. Increased Objectivity

Clearly the most attractive feature of meta-analysis is that it provides a new methodology for quantitative summary of previous research, in contrast to traditional narrative research reviews. The fallacious procedures of the box score or vote count methods of review are thus avoided. Note also that this approach generally reduces the various other sources of reviewer bias, although it is doubtful that any reviewing technique currently available could totally eliminate such bias. There is some probable advantage in that at least meta-analysis makes the biases, if any, more public.

2. Improved Perspective

The method of computing effect sizes that are aggregated across a series of studies provides an important opportunity for a vastly improved perspective in viewing an area of research. The more extensive and the more complex the research, the more this is true. For example, Smith and Glass (1977) included nearly 400 studies in their meta-analysis of psychotherapy outcome studies, a feat that was relatively simple for them, but generally regarded as prohibitive for a narrative review.

Furthermore, it is possible to compare studies across numerous characteristics, such as subject variables (like age, gender, IQ, and education), type of outcome measure, experimental design, degree of rigor, form of publication, and so on, as independent variables, creating an opportunity for genuinely new insights. For example, Smith and Glass (1977) were able to draw conclusions not reached by previous reviewers, namely, not only that psychotherapy works, but that it works almost equally well with all techniques.

The effect size is itself one of the features that most facilitates comparisons across studies. By converting all outcomes to a common metric, essentially based on standard deviation units, "scale-free" comparisons are feasible, that is, independent of any arbitrary units of measurement in the original reports.

Similarly, comparisons of effectiveness between different measurement techniques are equally feasible, which could easily point the way to the best choice of measures in future studies. Smith and Glass (1977), in another pertinent example, classified studies by degree of "reactivity" of dependent variables, a rating of the objectivity, or susceptibility to expectancy effects and test-taking attitude, likely to be reflected in the outcome measures. Although several descriptive variables showed low positive correlations with effect size (e.g., IQ of clients, similarity of therapists and clients), the highest correlation with effect size was shown by the reactivity measure ($r = .30$, $p<.01$).

This not only confirmed the wisdom of including the reactivity measure in the first place, but also made it possible to avoid a potentially serious source of bias in a simple manner. Hopefully, this communicated an important message to future researchers in choosing measures for use as dependent variables in similar studies.

3. Improved Recommendations for Future Research

As noted above, the box score or vote-counting methods of research review consistently underestimate the degree of demonstrated effect in a series of studies. Consequently, reviewers using traditional methods are more likely to miss proven effects and therefore make the erroneous recommendation that "more research is necessary," when in fact the phenomenon or treatment effect might be well established in the existing literature. If such is the case, then the obvious recommendation should be to expand and extend existing knowledge, not conduct one more indirect replication. There is already too much in good science that is "inefficient" (especially within the context of time and fiscal constraints) to warrant this unnecessary replication. These points are made more fully by Cooper and Rosenthal (1980) and Cooper (1989).

4. Specification of Studies

Meta-analyses, from the beginning, have evolved a consistent tradition of clearly specifying which studies were included in the meta-analysis and by what criteria. In some ways, this is a somewhat necessary result of the quantitative process itself, and in some ways it is simply a healthy (but fortuitous) characteristic of meta-analyses, that is, more tradition than absolute necessity. Whatever the reason, this represents an important step, since narrative reviewers in the past were typically likely to exclude studies simply on the basis of a vague, often unspecified, quality judgment that could simply be reviewer bias in disguise. Note that there is no rule preventing reviewer bias in meta-analysis, but it is less likely to occur.

One important question raised by this consideration is whether or not to exclude any studies solely on the basis of quality judgment. Smith and Glass (1977) solved the problem by including all studies that had at least an untreated control group or another therapy group (quite a qualitative step, actually), regardless of other indicators of rigor. At least two indices of internal validity were then included in their list of descriptive variables, permitting safe conclusions quite independent of rigor. This approach is the one that we too have chosen. In our opinion, it is justifiable (1) whenever the area of review includes a reasonable mixture of studies with high, medium, and low rigor, and (2) the methods and criteria for dealing with the question are entirely explicit. Indeed, Landman and Dawes (1982) repeated the Smith and Glass (1977) meta-analysis using only those studies that met minimum requirements of methodological quality and came to the same conclusions reached by Smith and Glass.

Conversely, if *all* (or nearly all) of the studies in an area of review are of low rigor, then no method of review or selection will place the reviewer on firm ground -- save only to point out the sorry state of research in the area.

5. *More Complete Data*

As Fiske (1983) points out, the process of meta-analysis forces the reviewer to focus more carefully on more aspects of all of the studies. It is a distinct result of the inherently quantitative nature of the meta-analysis, and it clearly illustrates the fundamental superiority of aggregating a large set of data, as opposed to a large set of narrative statements. Is it meaningful to combine all of the studies of neurotic (or whatever) patients, or are they too heterogeneous? What are the meaningful independent variables that can permit important comparisons? Do two measures sample the same or different constructs? What can or should be combined, and what can or should be compared? These questions are not answered quickly, but only after a detailed examination of all of the studies, which is a tedious but potentially highly significant process.

6. *Sharpening the Scientific Process*

It is more than slightly disconcerting to see how often the most basic information is omitted from primary reports. Authors frequently forget to include simple data such as the number of male and female subjects, mean age, educational level, and other subject data that should *always* be routinely reported. Broader use of meta-analysis should increase awareness of these problems and hopefully help to eliminate them.

Lastly, the realization that any single experiment is but one in a series of similar experiments should have a healthy impact on our view of the role of experiments, as well as the role of research reviews.

When is Meta-analysis Appropriate?

Any research question for which there are two or more studies could be reviewed by means of meta-analysis. One could profitably summarize the results of two studies in some circumstances with some gain in quantification at least. In actual practice, it is probably recommended when the number of studies exceeds 5 to 6, depending on the level of complexity. The only requirement is that the studies be addressed to a common question or hypothesis. So-called "outcome" studies (i.e., any studies testing the effectiveness or outcome of a treatment technique) are common and appropriate examples, but any group of studies with measured treatment effects could qualify.

It stands to reason that at least some of the studies in the identified group must be rigorously designed and conducted. No method presently available, nor likely in the future, will protect the reviewer from unwarranted conclusions based on a group of studies that are consistently faulty. The caveat "garbage in -- garbage out" is as true today as ever, and the introduction of the technique of meta-analysis has not changed this in any manner whatsoever. Similarly, it is reasonable to require that the studies to be reviewed be addressed to the same construct, even though different measures might be employed, or at least addressed to similar constructs that can be grouped at some more generic level of comparison.

In the present work, however, we have elected to develop a separate meta-analysis for studies of the effect of aerobic fitness training on (1) mood, (2) depression and anxiety, (3) self-concept, and (4) personality traits. These are distinct constructs, and, although anything can be combined if one wishes to become generic enough, nothing special is gained thereby in this instance. Supporting this view is the corresponding notion that these constructs are ordered on a continuum of permanence, with moods being the most evanescent or short-lived and personality traits the most enduring.

It would also seem to be obvious that "psychotherapy," as a treatment to be studied, is much more heterogeneous (i.e., more sharply divided between schools of thought on how best to proceed) than "aerobic fitness training" and therefore much more in need of combination of effects across diverse dependent variables in order to establish any effect at all. Aerobic fitness training, as a treatment to be studied, has the advantage that certain effects have already been well established (e.g., oxygen uptake, cardiovascular efficiency, low fat weight; see chapter 2), and consequently we are no longer asking the question of whether it has effects on anything.

How to Do a Meta-analysis

After addressing the questions of which studies to include, by what criteria, and so on, the actual process of doing a meta-analysis is relatively simple, especially if the number of studies reviewed is modest, say, around 25. Admittedly, however, it can be a tedious job if the studies number 200 to 400 or more, especially since most of the decision processes cannot at present be carried out by any automated machine language. Most reviewers with experience in the procedures for meta-analysis note that it can be a relatively time-consuming task, since no other reviewing process requires that they read entire reports so carefully! Also, the neophyte meta-analyst should be alerted to the fact that there have been some revisions in procedures, and hence the precise methods employed in the early works should not be applied uncritically in any meta-analysis initiated today.

The single most essential requirement for any meta-analysis is some quantitative measure of effect size. The first such use reported in a meta-analysis (Smith and Glass, 1977) was simply the difference between the means of the experimental and control groups, divided by the standard deviation of the control group. The resulting effect size is therefore expressed in standard deviation units which are scale free and can therefore be interpreted across studies.

For example, an effect size of 1.00 means that the difference between the experimental and control groups is equal to one standard deviation, or, more precisely, that the mean of the experimental group exceeds 84% of the values in the control group. (The reader will recall that 84% of the scores on the so-called normal curve fall below the value of the mean plus one standard deviation, whereas 16% of the scores lie above this value.) Correspondingly, an effect size of -1.00 would have the opposite meaning (84% of the values in the control group exceed the mean of the experimental group), whereas an effect size near 0.00 would mean that there is essentially no difference between groups. Thus, the observed effects in two or more studies can be compared, regardless of differences in measures, procedures, and so forth.

The effect sizes from a number of studies can then be used as the raw data in subsequent analyses. For example, in many instances, it will only be necessary to show that the mean effect size is greater than zero, meaning that the studies as grouped showed overall a significant net effect of the treatment under review.

Problems and Solutions in Meta-analysis

Given the potentially enormous social impact of the original Smith and Glass (1977) report (that psychotherapy is effective, and that all forms are about equally so), a vigorous response in the literature was totally predictable and in fact occurred in a short time.

The biggest concerns expressed by critics of the Smith and Glass (1977) approach were that (1) studies of both high and low rigor were included as equal contributors in the analysis, (2) effect sizes were computed for all reported dependent variables, yielding in some cases multiple non-independent effect sizes from some studies and therefore biasing the total effect size, and (3) the formula for computing effect size had no correction for sample size, and hence studies of small groups were included equally with studies of larger groups.

The first two concerns, that they included studies of low rigor and allowed multiple nonindependent effect sizes, have since been aptly addressed by Landman and Dawes

(1982) and Shapiro and Shapiro (1982); Smith and Glass *also* dealt with these problems. It is important to note that Landman and Dawes reached the same conclusion as Smith and Glass, even after eliminating all studies of low rigor and controlling for nonindependence of effect sizes.

The third concern, that the formula used for computing effect sizes was itself biased, needs some scrutiny at this point. In a most sobering statement, Hedges and Olkin (1985) have summarized their view of the magnitude of statistical problems in earlier meta-analyses:

> In this vein we note that many of the hundreds of research syntheses conducted to date use statistical procedures that are of questionable validity or are demonstrably incorrect. The conclusions of these meta-analyses may indeed be correct, but the statistical reasoning in support of these conclusions is not. (p. 14)

It is both disconcerting and ironic to discover that the technique of meta-analysis, developed almost solely as a means of increasing the quantitative nature of research reviews, has itself been the object of diverse subjective opinion. For example, the original Smith and Glass formula for computing effect sizes has been the subject of much discussion and revision, such that the original equation has little left to its advantage, except perhaps simplicity in logic and calculation, plus a degree of standardization and consistency.

Hedges (1981, 1982; see also Hedges & Olkin, 1985) has shown that the Smith and Glass method of dividing by the standard deviation of the control group introduces a bias that can and should be corrected. Dividing by the standard deviation of the control group, although justifiable in principle for consistency, will tend to overestimate effect sizes in small samples. Furthermore, the Smith and Glass formula is not strictly appropriate when there are both pre- and posttest data for experimental and control groups.

For these reasons, the formula (1), given in Appendix A, was used in this book to compute effect sizes (ES). This formula was used to provide a method of correcting for initial selection effects, since the pretest means for both the experimental and control groups were subtracted from the posttest means of each group. The correction was judged to be necessary in view of the large number of studies of aerobic fitness effects with selection problems, that is, nonrandom (self-selected) assignment to experimental and control groups. No algebraic correction can fully eliminate the problems of less rigorous designs; however it is still deemed to be a partial solution. In studies with random assignment to groups, the pretest mean of the experimental group should roughly equal the pretest mean of the control group, thus making the correction negligible when not necessary, but of some value with initially unequal groups.

Similarly, the small sample constant K in formula (3) approaches unity with increases in sample size, making the correction again negligible when not necessary. The reader who wishes a more detailed presentation of the burgeoning statistics of meta-analysis is referred to Hedges and Olkin (1985), Rosenthal (1984), and Rosenthal and Rubin (1986).

In studies where means and standard deviations were not fully reported, but statistics such as t, F, chi-square, or U, were given, the alternative formulae for calculating ES described by Glass et al. (1981, pp. 126-136; see also Cooper, 1989, pp. 101-105) were used.

Remaining Problems in Meta-analysis

As a final note, it should be mentioned that other methodological problems do exist. One of the most troublesome notions is that the experiments that have appeared in the literature might perhaps represent a bias in favor of only those studies that produced positive results. Presumably, those with negative results, potentially as many as 95% of the experiments (those that did not erroneously reject the null hypothesis), lie unpublished in the experimenter's office; that is, the so-called "file drawer problem." Rosenthal (1979) has shown that in many cases the actual number of studies lying unpublished in file drawers would necessarily have to reach unrealistically large numbers, suggesting that the published studies could not practically be the 5% that erroneously rejected the null hypothesis.

However, Bangert-Drowns (1986) has reported that "effect sizes from published articles are consistently higher than those found in dissertations" (p. 397). Although this might reflect the experience level of experimenters or possibly some other agent, it still raises the possibility that published studies might harbor some bias favoring those that rejected the null hypothesis erroneously (Type I error). It is especially troublesome here, because, for reasons of archival accessibility, it was necessary to exclude esoteric studies from the analysis. Thus, instead of reaching conclusions on the general nature of the effects of aerobic fitness training, we felt compelled to limit ourselves to summarizing the results of all publicly accessed experiments on aerobic fitness training, rather than all experiments, published or not.

Our primary reason for this position was to insure repeatability. Bullock and Svyantek (1985) have demonstrated rather dramatically that, under some circumstances, it can be impossible to replicate the results of a published meta-analysis. In our judgment, this is not due to an inherent shortcoming in the method itself, but rather it is a problem that may be encountered whenever the critical details of the meta-analysis are not reported, or if the original reports are not accessible. For example, if one finds (as did Bullock and Svyantek) a reported meta-analysis that omits such information as (1) the list of studies included, (2) the specific system for coding each study, and (3) the coded results for each study, then it should hardly come as a great surprise that the results cannot be repeated. The same can be said if the report includes a number of studies that subsequent investigators may find impossible to obtain for reasons of accessibility.

It is precisely for these reasons that we have elected to limit ourselves to studies that can be obtained through archival sources (no heroic efforts) and to summarize the coded results of each study in some detail as described in chapter 5.

Summary

As a summary of the logic and method of meta-analysis, we have emphasized the following points in the preceding chapter:

1. Questions dealt with in this chapter include (1) how and when did meta-analysis originate, (2) what are the primary strengths and benefits of meta-analysis, (3) when is it most appropriate, and (4) are there unsolved problems in using this technique?

2. The nature of scientific evidence was discussed, with emphasis on the differences between primary and secondary reports of research. The relative importance of each source was discussed.

3. Characteristics of traditional narrative research reviews were examined in some detail. Several consistent sources of error commonly exist in so-called box score or vote counting methods of reviewing primary reports.

4. Meta-analysis, originally introduced as an objective alternative to traditional narrative reviews, was reviewed.

5. The most important strengths and benefits of meta-analysis as enumerated in this discussion were:

    a. Increased objectivity
    b. Improved perspective
    c. Improved recommendations for future research
    d. Specification of studies
    e. More complete data
    f. Sharpening the scientific process

6. Consideration was given to the question of when it is best to do a meta-analysis. In general, it is appropriate whenever there are a modest number of studies addressed to the same or similar constructs, with at least some of the studies being rigorously designed.

7. The process of conducting a meta-analysis is relatively simple, although it can become tedious with large numbers of studies. Actual computation of

effect sizes (ES) is straightforward and has a number of advantages.

8. Some early concerns with meta-analyses were (1) that studies of both high and low rigor were included as equal partners, (2) that multiple ESs were computed from single studies yielding biased total effect sizes, and (3) that the initial formulae used to compute ESs failed to correct for small sample size. Each of these concerns has since been remedied.

9. Specific formulae used in the present meta-analysis were described and explained.

10. Some remaining problems were discussed, most notably the unsolved question of biased differences between published and unpublished primary reports in an area.

11. Additional problems may occur because of (1) incomplete reporting of important details in a specific meta-analysis, or (2) by including studies that are not otherwise available through archival sources. To avoid these problems, this book is limited to studies that can be obtained without resorting to heroic efforts, and the coded results of each study are carefully summarized. In this manner, the present report is considered to be highly replicable.

FIVE

SEARCH METHODS

The purpose of this chapter is to outline the literature search methods used in preparation for the research review to be presented in subsequent chapters. How were specific reports chosen over all of those available, and how were the data from each report summarized? What were the primary and secondary library resources that were most helpful? Were computer assisted searches used, and with what result? Of critical importance, what criteria were developed for including versus excluding studies from the many examined? And what specific effect size (ES) calculations were made in each of the groupings to be reported? Finally, what planned comparisons were made, that is, how were studies regrouped for additional comparisons beyond those covered in the individual reports?

What and Where Is the Target Literature?

Research on the psychological effects of aerobic fitness training is clearly of significant interest to and of broad impact on an extremely diverse audience. Important examples include the public at large, the social, behavioral/psychological, and biological sciences, most of the specialties of the field of medicine, nursing, and health care, plus the fields of exercise physiology, education, sports and athletics, and substantial segments of business and industry. Small wonder then that the results of this research have appeared in an extremely broad array of journals, representing quite a number of disciplines. This fact alone may be regarded as somewhat intimidating, however, it strongly suggests that the literature search procedures must be broadly based and ultimately very time-consuming. We can testify that this initial expectation was more than borne out by our experiences. The full search for this project eventually extended over an active period of more than 8 months, with a less active period extending several years beyond.   The work included   two computer-assisted searches, the contribution of an extensive unpublished bibliography on psychological considerations on exercise, repeated trips to several major research libraries, hundreds of reprint post cards, and the persistent efforts of two world class librarians.

The following is a summary listing of the major search procedures employed, given in the chronological order   in which they were used.   Each method of search produced some number of finds, plus an even greater number of reports that eventually did not qualify for various reasons, with a larger number in the beginning and only a few remaining finds during the final search efforts.   Therefore, it is not practical to report which of the following search strategies produced the greatest number of finds.   There was a great deal of overlap, and of course we could have recorded how many independent times each find was in fact uncovered by each search strategy, but that would have been another project for another day.   As expected, however, no single source (no matter how extensive) produced all of the reports that qualified for this review.   To put it another way, every source consulted produced some new finds not reported by others.   This means that all previous bibliographic sources have some omissions, and also hints that others possibly were missed in this work.   This is not so much the fault of any bibliographic source, but rather an indicator of the breadth of   disciplines (and   journals) represented by investigators who have published reports on the   effects   of   fitness   training, not to mention the frequency with which additional reports appear.

Computer-Assisted Searches

The search was initiated with   a *Medline* computer search of the National Library of Medicine. Several subject categories were searched, including aerobic fitness, physical exercise, psychological test, questionnaire, mood, personality, self-concept, and lifestyle.   Although the result   was nearly overwhelming, it was still finite and therefore possible to review each resulting citation.   Reprint request post cards were used as the first effort to obtain copies of articles, plus photocopies of   articles   available   from journals in the library of the Naval Health Research Center (NHRC). Articles for which post cards were returned or which otherwise produced no response in 2 months were then requested by interlibrary loan. Since the *Medline* printout includes abstracts of recent articles, it was possible to identify a very substantial number of articles via this method. Articles for which there was no abstract were examined directly through library sources.

Next, a *Dialog* search of the *Psycinfo* database was conducted. This is a computer equivalent of *Psychological Abstracts*, that is, a search of the world's literature in psychology and related behavioral sciences. The search in this case was keyed on physical endurance, aerobic fitness, and various personality traits, including anxiety, depression, extraversion/introversion, and self-concept. This produced somewhat fewer articles than *Medline*, but still a substantial number, many of which were included.

Additional Search Methods

Sachs and Buffone (1985) have compiled an extensive unpublished bibliography of over 1300 references on "Psychological considerations in exercise, including exercise as psychotherapy, exercise addiction, and the psychology of running." A large number of these citations (e.g., those on addiction) are not directly relevant to this review; however, a significant number of finds were still made from this source, all of which were ordered through interlibrary loan or photocopied where available via other library sources.

In addition to collecting articles that qualified for the present review, a collection of review articles and book chapters was also acquired at the same time with quite extensive results. Some of these reviews are highly specialized in nature, but others are impressively comprehensive, current, and close in content to the intended target literature of this search. Those primary reviews that most closely fit these characteristics were Dishman (1985), Doan and Scherman (1987), Folkins and Sime (1981), Goff and Dimsdale (1985), Hughes (1984), Morgan and Goldston (1987), Sonstroem (1984), and Taylor, Sallis, and Needle (1985). Great care was taken to include every qualified article cited by any one of these reviewers, although in every case the decision to include an article was based on direct examination of the original report, rather than the reviewer's evaluative comments.

In addition, the following reviews were judged to be either less current or more specialized than those that most closely covered the intended target literature. The references cited were still evaluated carefully, with some positive results. These secondary source reviews were Ben-Schlomo and Short (1983), Blair (1984), Browne and Mahoney (1984), Buffone (1984), Cureton (1963), Dienstbier (1984), Dishman (1982), Dishman, Sallis, and Orenstein (1985), Greist et al. (1981), Hammett (1967), Haskell (1984), Howell and Alderman (1967), Layman (1974), Ledwidge (1980), Martin and Dubbert (1982), Mellion (1985), Mihevic (1982), Shephard (1985), Silva and Shultz (1984), Sime (1984), Stamler (1985), Tomporowski and Ellis (1986), and Weinstein and Meyers (1983). It should be noted that these reviews were consulted *in addition to* reviews cited in previous chapters, covering the literature on exercise and risk of coronary heart disease (chapter 1) and other health benefits (chapter 2).

By this point it was clear that a certain core group of journals accounted for a majority of the qualified articles, therefore a search of recent issues over the last three years was conducted to catch recently appearing articles not otherwise cited in any other source. Our goal was to include in the review all articles that appeared through 1988; however, the final search efforts were made in November, 1990, and consequently a number of articles that appeared in 1989 were located and included if otherwise qualified.

Lastly, the bibliographies of all qualified articles were scanned in a routine manner as copies were received, especially in cases where the article was quite recent or appeared in a relatively obscure (and potentially unique) source.

Since every search method produced some results, it is still assumed that some unknown number of articles were missed. Articles with brief ambiguous titles, that fail to mention in the abstract that they evaluated psychological effects of aerobic fitness training, and that were not cited by any other source, stood a very good chance of being missed. Fortunately, it is highly unlikely that a few missed articles would affect the outcome of the meta-analysis, unless there were some unknown systematic bias that lead to the exclusion of articles of a single type. We can only apologize here for any errors of omission.

Selection Criteria

Even though we were frequently surprised by the number of reports on various aspects of the effects of aerobic fitness training, we did not encounter any unanticipated characteristics in the reported research that necessitated revision of the selection criteria midway through the search. The following, then, were the selection criteria as used throughout the process:

1. *Intent to study aerobic fitness effects.* The investigators indicated that it was their intention to assess psychological changes produced by aerobic fitness training, rather than some similar-sounding, but unrelated investigation, such as measuring sport personality.

2. *Used standardized psychological test instrument.* By "psychological changes," we simply mean those measured by any standardized psychological test instrument that yields objective, numerical scores.

3. *Based on pre- and posttest comparisons.* Test instruments were administered in most studies in a pre- and posttest fashion. Exceptions were permitted, but noted in the subsequent planned comparisons.

4. *Aerobic fitness of subjects measured.* Some measure of aerobic fitness of the subjects was taken before and after the period of training. Studies in which the fitness measure was only implicit (provided that the fitness training regimen was otherwise plausible) were still included, but this procedural compromise was noted. Studies (or groups) in which no pre- to posttest improvements in fitness were found were not included. For example, in one study (Kowal, Patton, & Vogel, 1978), only the males showed significant improvements in fitness measures, whereas the females

showed no change, and consequently we included only the male group data in the meta-analysis.

5. *Fitness training within recommended guidelines.* By "aerobic fitness training," we mean any of the recommended rhythmic endurance exercises listed by the ACSM (1978, 1991) within guidelines for frequency, intensity, and duration (see chapter 2).   Most of the experiments reported using jogging/running as the exercise of choice; however, any other aerobic activity was accepted, especially since this raised possibilities for additional planned comparisons.

6. *Studies of effects in special groups.* Studies of special groups were common and quite welcome if the other criteria were met.   Examples were studies of fitness effects in depressed subjects, postmyocardial infarction patients, children, and the elderly.

7. *No selection based on merit alone.* No studies were dropped on the basis of quality or merit judgments, although there were tempting moments.   This decision was made in the beginning, partly in the belief that any study (no matter how poorly designed or conducted) may still serve as the impetus for important work in the future, and partly because we intuitively doubted our ability to draw a defensible line between "good" and "not good" studies. There is of course a significant literature that has borne out this intuition (Cooper, 1989, pp. 63-68).   It must be remembered that a study that is not rigorously designed is not necessarily incorrect in its findings, although it may by itself be ambiguous, and it may or may not ultimately be shown to be correct.   Thus, instead of an a priori decision to omit studies on quality grounds, we prefer the strategy adopted by Smith and Glass (1977).   These authors included all identifiable studies, regardless of quality, but they also compared effect sizes of high and low rigor studies.   In this manner, there is utterly no sacrifice or increased risk of unfounded conclusions, in exchange for a more fully comprehensive coverage of what in fact has been reported in the literature.

Characteristics of Studies Not Included

There were of course reasons other than quality that served as the basis for excluding some studies that otherwise seemed superficially relevant, or very nearly so. In other words, there were some studies that met all of the criteria listed above, but that were still excluded. The major reasons for not including closely-related studies were the following:

1. *Nonstandardized dependent variables.* The investigators used a nonstandardized measure as the dependent variable. Examples included interviews, unpublished self-rating scales, and projective techniques (e.g., inkblots and figure drawings) with subjective or otherwise nonreproducible scoring methods.

2. *Nonaerobic exercise.* The exercise was clearly not aerobic (e.g., weightlifting) and the investigators had no stated intention of measuring aerobic fitness.

3. *Studies of sport personality.* Studies of the so-called "sport personality" were not included. These studies are generally surveys of athletic temperament (Eysenck, Nias, & Cox, 1982), with no intent to measure aerobic fitness per se. Studies in which endurance athletes served as subjects and which otherwise met our criteria were included.

4. *Dissertations and theses.* The decision to omit dissertations and theses was a relatively painful one, since Sachs and Buffone (1985) list 140 dissertations and theses, and the *Psycinfo* search result included 28 dissertations. We judged, however, that an abstract alone is not sufficient for a review of the present nature, and the cost of purchasing full photocopies (often $30 to 50 per dissertation) was not feasible. We also determined early in the search that, to maximize the replicability of our meta-analysis, we would include only archival reports that could be obtained through reasonable effort by a conscientious and professional reviewer with average-to-good resources. In other words, a meta-analysis that could only be repeated or extended through heroic effort and unlimited resources

is virtually unreplicable, a consequence that we elected to avoid.

5. *Studies reported in abstract form only.* We did not accept any studies reported in abstract form only. Proceedings of professional meetings were the most frequent example.

6. *Nonarchival reports.* Studies that were reported only as nonarchival (i.e., not available in any major research library or computer search) technical reports were not included. These reports are often not refereed, however, the decision not to include was based solely on the fact that any nonarchival report will presumably be unavailable for anyone wishing to repeat our work.

7. *Foreign language reports.* Lastly, foreign language reports were excluded. This decision was not anticipated, but was ultimately unavoidable because of the consistent exclusion of such studies in our search sources. We can only acknowledge this shortcoming with sincere apologies.

Coding Methods

The coding summary duplicated in Appendix A was used for each study included in our meta-analysis. Each summary thus provided the information necessary for calculation of effect sizes, plus other characteristics used for additional planned comparisons.

Effect sizes were calculated for each reported dependent variable. Thus, if the experimenters used a standardized scale with six subtests, and all of the necessary data were duly reported, then we calculated six effect sizes. If these same experimenters also included a second inventory with 13 subtests, then we also calculated the additional 13 effect sizes. At no time, however, did more than one effect size from one study enter into any one meta-analysis.

Although this might seem to be an excessive number of effect sizes, it was our judgment that we had no alternative in a review of this nature, *provided*, however, that we were able to make comparisons in such a manner that each study contributed only one effect size to each meta-analysis.   For example, consider an experiment in which the investigators wished to study the effects of aerobic fitness training on mood states, certainly not an unusual project, and they chose the POMS (Profile of Mood States) as their primary dependent variable, again not at all unusual.   The POMS, however, consists of six subtests that yield six scores (tension, depression, anger, vigor, fatigue, and confusion), with no item overlap.   Even though the six resulting effect sizes could be summed or averaged, it is our position that this is both unnecessary and less efficient in the present meta-analysis, since there is an *a priori* basis for predicting that some mood scores (e.g., vigor) will likely change more than others (e.g., confusion) as a result of aerobic fitness training.   Summing all scores can indicate if there was an effect "on anything" in the realm of mood, which of course may still be justified in specific experiments, but not in this work.

We thus concluded that it would be more meaningful to conduct six meta-analyses in this case, keeping strictly at the level of the most meaningful constructs, and enabling us to draw conclusions about the effects of aerobic fitness training on each of the six mood scores.   In this manner, each individual study contributed only one effect size to each meta-analysis, thus controlling for the problem of nonindependence of effect sizes discussed above in connection with the report by Smith and Glass (1977).   It also allowed us to keep those studies in which the investigators reported only a portion of the total number of scores, because they would have been discarded if we had chosen to compare studies on the basis of total change scores alone.   There is of course the risk that unreported subtest scores were in fact not significant, meaning that those reported were actually a biased subsample of the total number of scores.   This is a problem to which we return.

Setting aside these particular problems for the moment, our overall approach is feasible whenever there are a number of studies that use the same measure as the dependent variable, clearly one of the advantages of limiting this analysis to studies that used standardized tests (such as the POMS in the example cited).   This in turn necessitated further safeguards against Type I errors resulting from the increased number of comparisons. It also presupposes a body of research on a treatment where it is already established that there is an effect "on anything." Otherwise, summing into total scores is more meaningful in such early stages.

Information in the Coding Summary

The coding summary (see Appendix A) of each study included information about the test groups, experimental design, measure of aerobic fitness, fitness training protocol, and the independent and dependent variables.

1. Test Groups
Studies were grouped on the basis of the primary constructs measured by the dependent variables. The test groups, created on an *a posteriori* basis, were (1) mood, (2) self-concept, and (3) personality. It was quickly determined, however, that a large number of the studies in the mood group were focused only on depression and anxiety, and therefore an additional group was identified for separate meta-analysis of these studies. If a report included more than one test instrument, and this was not unusual, then more than one coding summary was prepared for that report.

2. Experimental Design
All studies were classified by type of design, using the framework and terminology used by Campbell and Stanley (1966). This allowed us to group studies by level of rigor, for example, pre-experimental (which we term "survey studies"), quasi-experimental, and true experimental designs, in order to test for differences in effect sizes between studies that differed in rigor. Such comparisons were highly essential, since, as described above, studies were included in the meta-analysis regardless of our opinion or rating of experimental rigor. Only by doing the former is the latter justified.

3. Measure of Aerobic Fitness
This information was deemed to be necessary, because (as described in chapter 2) there are a number of measures

of aerobic fitness (such as treadmill, bicycle ergometer, step test), plus various protocols, maximum versus sub-maximum endurance tests, and so on. In this manner, we could determine whether or not there were differences in effect sizes by measure of fitness. If there were no such differences by measure of fitness, then such a finding might suggest that experimenters can feel free to choose any one of a number of measures on the basis of convenience, cost, personal experience, training, or whatever. Should the opposite be found, then perhaps some fitness measures would be less recommended for future work in this area. This information also permitted comparisons across test groups for possible interaction effects: for example, it is conceivable that fitness training affects mood regardless of fitness measure, whereas effects on personality traits are only observed under certain conditions.

4. Fitness Training Protocol

Recorded here was the kind of activity (running, biking, swimming, etc.), plus information on duration, intensity, frequency, and length of time in the program. Obviously, a number of potentially provocative comparisons were possible on the basis of these data. For example, do running, biking, and swimming all produce similar effects, or do they differ in some respect? Do these differences (if any) hold at all levels of training? Are there differences between studies that followed ACSM guidelines for minimum fitness training versus those that did not? Are there significant interactions? The potential for new insights here was judged to be considerable.

5. Independent Variables

The information coded here is generally self-evident. The independent variable was most often given by the names of the experimental groups -- depressed clients, postmyocardial infarction patients, athletes, and so on -- beyond the fitness training procedure itself. Again, a number of provocative comparisons were possible on the basis of information between controls and patient groups, males versus females, various age groups, and so on, plus the added question of possible interaction effects.

6. *Dependent Variables*

This information is self-explanatory and follows from the information given above on calculation of effect sizes. Wherever possible, preference was given to calculating effect sizes by formula (1) as described in chapter 4. Values from significance tests (t, F, chi-square, etc.) were included only when it was not possible to calculate effect size by formula (1).

Summary

The search, selection, and coding procedures contained the following major components:

1. The target literature (as well as the target audience) for research on the psychological effects of aerobic fitness training is unusually broad, and cuts across a number of disciplines. As a result, any literature search on this topic must be equally broad.
2. The methods in this case included two computer-assisted searches, visual search of approximately two dozen journals that comprised the core group in this area, and detailed use of the reference list of other articles, reviews, and an extensive unpublished bibliography.
3. Selection criteria for studies included:

    a. Specifically directed at effects of aerobic fitness training.
    b. Used standardized test instrument as the dependent variable.
    c. Included both pre- and posttest measures, with exceptions noted.
    d. Some measure of aerobic fitness taken, with plausible exceptions noted.
    e. Aerobic fitness training within guidelines of the ACSM (1978, 1991).
    f. No restriction on subjects, such as age, sex, medical status, prior fitness level, etc.
    g. Studies of both high and low apparent design quality, but with later ratings of rigor.

4. Characteristics of studies NOT included:

   a. Nonstandard measure as the dependent variable.
   b. Exercise clearly not aerobic.
   c. Studies of "sport personality."
   d. Reports not accessible from general research archives including dissertations and theses, studies reported in abstract form only, nonarchival technical reports, and foreign language reports.

5. Data from selected studies were summarized by coding:

   a. Grouping by tests/constructs measured.
   b. Experimental design.
   c. Measure of aerobic fitness.
   d. Fitness training protocol.
   e. Independent variables studied.
   f. Dependent variables reported.

6. Studies within test groups were combined such that only one effect size from one study contributed to one meta-analysis, rather than an alternate summing method.

7. A number of additional planned comparisons were described, including subject variables (age, sex, etc.) grouped under the independent variable.

SIX

MOOD STUDIES

This chapter is a review of the studies of the effects of aerobic fitness training on mood state. Mood is usually defined as an individual's feelings or affective status at a specific moment, hence it often refers to a temporary state, as opposed to a trait, generally agreed to be a more enduring characteristic. Questionnaires that are designed to measure mood states will usually indicate as much in the instructions to subjects; subjects are instructed to respond in terms of how they feel at the present time, for example, "now," "today," or "in the last week."

Moods are therefore the most transient of the psychological characteristics to be reviewed in the present work, and presumably also the most responsive to treatment effects in a fitness training group, especially as compared to more stable characteristics such as self-concept and fundamental personality traits. Intuitively, one might expect to find the largest effect sizes to be shown on mood questionnaires, but only at the cost that such responses would be the most easily influenced by response sets, such as acquiescence or suggestion, which are generally termed expectancy effects.

The mood studies reviewed in this chapter are those in which the investigators evaluated mood in a relatively broad sense in normal subjects, and therefore we have *temporarily* excluded all studies in which the primary purpose was to evaluate the effect of fitness training on depression and anxiety, especially in subjects who show such clinical symptoms at a problem level. In the more broadly-based group of studies, the intent was to evaluate mood in general, which is the subject of this chapter. There is a second group of studies, in which the intent was to evaluate depression and anxiety specifically as an indication of the *therapeutic* value of aerobic fitness training; these studies are reviewed in chapter 7. This distinction is only partly conceptual and partly a matter of convenience. A final integration of the two sets of findings will be necessary in a later chapter, and we apologize for any temporary confusion.

Measures of Mood State

Two standardized tests have been used in the studies of effects on mood: the Profile of Mood States (POMS), and the Multiple Affect Adjective Check List (MAACL). Both of these instruments met our requirements for being included in the present review, and they also have the added advantage that both have been used extensively in research on mood states, both in fitness studies and in a host of other areas.

POMS

The POMS (McNair, Lorr, & Droppleman, 1971) consists of 65 adjectives rated on a 5-point scale from "not at all" to "extremely." Subjects are instructed to respond in terms of how they have felt during the past week "including today." There are six nonoverlapping scales: tension, depression, anger, vigor, fatigue, and confusion. The test has the advantage that it can be administered quickly (about ten minutes), and few subjects have difficulty with the materials. It has been well reviewed by Eichman (1978) who concluded that the "POMS appears to have no peer" (p. 1018), as well as Weckowicz (1978) whose observations were similarly positive.

MAACL

The MAACL (Zuckerman and Lubin, 1965) consists of 132 adjectives. Subjects are instructed to check only those words that describe their feelings. The scale is thus open-ended with regard to the total number of adjectives checked. There are two forms of the test which differ only in instruction, the "today" form and the "in general" form. There are three nonoverlapping scales: anxiety, depression, and hostility. The test can usually be administered in about five minutes.

Both Kelly (1972) and Megargee (1972) express concern about the development procedures and validity of the MAACL, as well as the fact that scores show correlations with various measures of response set, such as social desirability and acquiescence or expectancy.

Independent Variables

There were 26 studies identified that constitute the mood group. Each study was given an identification number alphabetically by author. The 26 studies, including identification number, authors, year of publication, and mood scale used (POMS or MAACL), are listed in Table 6.1. Specific design characteristics of the POMS studies and the MAACL studies are summarized in Table 6.2 (a and b, respectively).

Each table gives the following for each study in the mood group: identification number of each publication, number of groups reported and/or used in the meta-analysis, number of subjects in the experimental and control groups, number of male and female subjects, mean age of subjects, experimental design and type of effect size (explained below), fitness exercise, and measure(s) of fitness.

This information is relatively self-explanatory, with the exception of experimental design and type of effect size. Each of these entries in Table 6.2 is actually a rating of the study as reported. The experimental design ratings were based on the list provided by Campbell and Stanley (1966), and consist of the following designs:

Pre-experimental designs
1. One-shot case study
2. One group pretest and posttest
3. Static group comparison

True experimental designs
4. Pretest-posttest control group
5. Solomon four-group
6. Posttest-only control group

Quasi-experimental designs
7. Time series experiment
8. Equivalent time samples
9. Equivalent materials samples
10. Nonequivalent control group
11. Counterbalanced designs
12. Separate-sample pretest-posttest

Table 6.1. Mood group, showing identification number,
authors, year of publication, and scale used.

ID	Authors	Year	Scale
1M	Berger and Owen	1983	POMS
2M	Blumenthal, Schocken, Needels, and Hindle	1982	POMS
3M	Blumenthal, Williams, Needels, and Wallace	1982	POMS
4M	Carney, McKevitt, Goldberg, Hagberg, Delmez, and Harter	1983	MAACL
5M	Folkins	1976	MAACL
6M	Folkins, Lynch, and Gardner	1972	MAACL
7M	Frazier and Nagy	1989	POMS
8M	Goldberg, Hagberg, Delmez, Carney, McKevitt, Ehsani, and Harter	1980	MAACL
9M	Gondola and Tuckman	1982	POMS
10M	Gondola and Tuckman	1983	POMS
11M	Johnson, Collins, Higgins, Harrington, Connolly, Dolphin, McCreery, Brady, and O'Brien	1985	POMS
12M	Kowal, Patton, and Vogel	1978	POMS
13M	McDonald, Beckett, and Hodgdon	1991	POMS
14M	Morgan, O'Connor, Ellickson, and Bradley	1988	POMS

(table continues)

(Table 6.1, continued)

ID	Authors	Year	Scale
15M	Morgan, O'Connor, Sparling, and Pate	1987	POMS
16M	Morgan and Pollock	1977	POMS
17M	Moses, Steptoe, Mathews, and Edwards	1989	POMS
18M	Nagy and Frazier	1988	POMS
19M	Perri and Templer	1984-85	MAACL
20M	Rudy and Estok	1983	MAACL
21M	Simons and Birkimer	1988	POMS
22M	Steptoe, Edwards Moses, and Mathews	1989	POMS
23M	Suominen-Troyer, Davis, Ismail, and Salvendy	1986	MAACL
24M	Wilfley and Kunce	1986	POMS
25M	Williams and Getty	1986	POMS
26M	Young	1979	MAACL

Table 6.2. Design characteristics of the mood group.

Study	No. of Groups	Ne	Nc	Nm	Nf	Age	Design/ ES-type	Fitness Exercise	Measure of Fitness
						a. POMS Studies			
1M	2+	33	42	31	44	22.3	10/1	swimming	compulsory class
2M	2	15	11	--	--	69.3	2/3	bike	BP, HR, Wt
3M	2	16	16	10	22	45.1	10/3	walk/jog	BP, HR, Wt
7M	2	31	55	--	86	21.4	10/1	dance	class completion
9M-M	1m	280	--	280	--	32	3/4	marathon	running history
9M-F	1f	--	68	--	68	34	3/4	marathon	running history
10M-A	2	68	186	--	254	30?	3/3	marathon	running history
10M-B	2	210	186	--	396	30?	3/3	10km	running history
11M	1	6	--	6	--	21	2/4	cycling	%BF, VO2max
12M	1	85	--	85	--	20?	2/4	basic training	%BF, VO2max
13M	1	92	--	--	--	27.7	1/3	military training	VO2max
14M	1	14	--	14	--	26.4	1/4	running history	running history
15M	1	15	--	--	15	27.2	1/4	running history	running history
16M	1	27	--	27	--	24.8	1/4	elite runners	VO2max
17M	2	18	18	11	25	38.8	4/2	walk/jog	12-min run

(table continues)

(Table 6.2, continued)

Study	No. of Groups	Ne	Nc	Nm	Nf	Age	Design/ ES-type	Fitness Exercise	Measure of Fitness
18M	2	31	54	--	85	21.4	3/2	dance	exercise history
21M	2	54	75	52	77	43.5	10/1	walk/jog	HR
22M	2	17	16	5	28	37.0	10/1	walk/run	bike ergometer
24M	2	49	34	--	--	43.0	10/2	walk/run	lap run, HR
25M	2	266	40	--	--	20?	10/1	jog/dance	class completion

b. MAACL Studies

Study	No. of Groups	Ne	Nc	Nm	Nf	Age	Design/ ES-type	Fitness Exercise	Measure of Fitness
4M	2	4	4	6	2	40?	4/1	bike/jog	VO2max
5M	2	18	18	36	0	50?	4/3	walk/jog	BP, HR, lipids
6M	2	42	42	42	42	19?	10/1	jog	HR, 1.75-m run
8M	1	4	0	3	1	33	2/2	jog/bike walk	VO2max
19M	2	23	19	14	28	65.4	10/1	walk/jog	compulsory class
20M	1	319	0	0	319	35?	1/3	10k/ marathon	running history
23M	2	10	20	--	30	42.6	10/2	run/jog	HR, BP, BF
26M	2	16	16	16	16	30+	10/1	jog	HR, BP, %LBW

Note: Ne and Nc = number of subjects in the experimental and control groups; Nm and Nf = number of male and female subjects; Age = mean for the total group; BP = blood pressure, HR = heart rate Wt = body weight, %BF = percent body fat, %LBW = percent lean body weight.

13. Separate-sample pretest-posttest control group
14. Multiple time series
15. Recurrent institutional cycle
16. Regression-discontinuity

Although this system does not include all possible experimental designs, it does include all of those encountered in this analysis. The ratings of design do not constitute either an interval or an ordinal scale, but rather they are a nominal system for categorizing studies, so that, for example, planned comparisons between surveys or pre-experiments (i.e., studies with a nominal design rating of 1-3) and experiments (true experiments and quasi-experiments with nominal design ratings of 4-16) could be made.

Studies with a nominal design rating of 1-3, which Campbell and Stanley termed pre-experiments, are hereafter referred to as survey studies. In each case these are studies that consisted of only one group and/or only posttest observations (with no pretest for comparison) and therefore no explicit independent variable. Although some of these studies were notably intensive efforts, all survey studies suffer the increased risk of confound effects on their results.

It also seemed possible that the method of calculating effect sizes could make a difference in results; therefore all effect sizes were rated from 1 to 4 in the following manner, in decreasing order of preference (the criterion when more than one method was possible):

1. The effect size was calculated by using the full formula described in chapter 4.
2. Effect size was calculated by the original Smith and Glass (1977) formula, based on the difference between two means divided by the standard deviation.
3. Where means and standard deviations were not reported, but statistics such as t, F, and chi-square were available, effect sizes were calculated by means of the formulae described by Cooper (1989, pp. 101-105).
4. Only one observation on one group was reported. but it was still possible to compare these scores

with published norms for the standardized test, that is, using normative data as the "control group."

In cases where the authors reported that the results were not significant, and they included no specific data from which to calculate effect sizes, an arbitrary effect size of 0.00 was assigned. Although this undoubtedly introduced some error, it was felt that excluding such reports would have introduced even greater error. Thus, the lesser (and more conservative) error was chosen.

Therefore, even though there was variability in the method of calculating effect sizes, it was possible to determine if this had any effect on the results of the meta-analysis by simply comparing effect sizes by method of calculation as one of the planned comparisons. Including studies of all experimental designs and methods of calculating effect sizes enabled us to include much more of the published data and also to determine whether or not our a priori concerns were justified. This in turn could have a significant effect on our ultimate interpretation of the findings in the area.

Results by Study

The standard normal deviate (Z) scores and effect sizes for each study in the mood group are given in Tables 6.3 and 6.4. Column headings for Tables 6.3 and 6.4 are as follows:

1. Study: Each study is listed by identification number, as in Table 6.1. Results for males and females are listed separately when this was included in the original report (studies 1M, 6M, 9M, and 26M). Different events (10 k and marathon) are listed separately in one case (10M).
2. Z: The standard normal deviate or Z score, derived in the usual manner.
3. ES: Effect size (ES) calculated by one of the four methods previously described. Negative ES = decrease in mean score for the experimental group on posttest relative to controls.

Table 6.3. Z scores and effect sizes as calculated for each study.*

Study	Z	ES	ES-m	ES-f	ES-ya	ES-ma	ES-ea	ES-sur	ES-exp

a. Tension Scores -- POMS Studies

Study	Z	ES	ES-m	ES-f	ES-ya	ES-ma	ES-ea	ES-sur	ES-exp
1M-M	-0.89	-0.351	-0.351		-0.351				-0.351
1M-F	-2.02	-0.651		-0.651	-0.651				-0.651
3M	-1.99	-0.794				-0.794			-0.794
7M	-0.36	-0.079		-0.079	-0.079				-0.079
9M-M	-3.70	-0.492	-0.492			-0.492		-0.492	
9M-F	-3.70	-0.366		-0.366		-0.366		-0.366	
10M-A	0.42	0.053		0.053		0.053		0.053	
10M-B	-2.03	-0.207		-0.207		-0.207		-0.207	
11M	-3.70	-0.587	-0.587		-0.587			-0.587	
12M	-1.96	-0.437	-0.437		-0.437			-0.437	
13M	-0.66	-0.139			-0.139			-0.139	
14M	-0.65	-0.373	-0.373		-0.373			-0.373	
15M	-0.81	-0.447		-0.447	-0.447			-0.447	
16M	-3.30	-0.358	-0.358		-0.358			-0.358	
17M	0.00	0.000				0.000			0.000
18M	-0.37	-0.082		-0.082	-0.082			-0.082	
21M	-1.83	-0.331				-0.331			-0.331
22M	-2.17	-0.830				-0.830			-0.830
24M	0.30	0.067				0.067			0.067
25M	-0.39	-0.044			-0.044				-0.044

b. Anger Scores -- POMS Studies

Study	Z	ES	ES-m	ES-f	ES-ya	ES-ma	ES-ea	ES-sur	ES-exp
1M-M	-2.39	-0.949	-0.949		-0.949				-0.949
1M-F	-0.95	-0.312		-0.312	-0.312				-0.312
2M	-2.02	-0.950					-0.950	-0.950	
3M	0.00	0.000				0.000			0.000
7M	0.00	-0.015		-0.015	-0.015				-0.015
9M-M	0.82	0.068	0.068			0.068		0.068	
9M-F	0.00	0.000		0.000		0.000		0.000	
10M-A	1.58	0.201		0.201		0.201		0.201	
10M-B	-0.42	-0.042		-0.042		-0.042		-0.042	
11M	-2.36	-0.256	-0.256		-0.256			-0.256	
12M	-0.41	-0.089	-0.089		-0.089			-0.089	
13M	-0.66	-0.139			-0.139			-0.139	
14M	-0.36	-0.205	-0.205		-0.205			-0.205	

(table continues)

(Table 6.3, continued)

Study	Z	ES	ES-m	ES-f	ES-ya	ES-ma	ES-ea	ES-sur	ES-exp
15M	-1.04	-0.575		-0.575	-0.575			-0.575	
16M	-2.60	-0.283	-0.283		-0.283			-0.283	
17M	0.00	0.000				0.000			0.000
18M	-0.40	-0.089		-0.089	-0.089			-0.089	
21M	-1.76	-0.321				-0.321			-0.321
22M	0.22	0.079				0.079			0.079
24M	0.85	0.191				0.191			0.191
25M	-1.19	-0.137			-0.137				-0.137

c. Depression Scores -- POMS Studies

Study	Z	ES	ES-m	ES-f	ES-ya	ES-ma	ES-ea	ES-sur	ES-exp
1M-M	-0.38	-0.141	-0.141		-0.141				-0.141
1M-F	-1.80	-0.580		-0.580	-0.580				-0.580
3M	-2.34	-0.944				-0.944			-0.944
7M	0.54	0.119		0.119	0.119				0.119
9M-M	-3.70	-0.354	-0.354			-0.354		-0.354	
9M-F	-3.70	-0.305		-0.305		-0.305		-0.305	
10M-A	1.03	0.130		0.130		0.130		0.130	
10M-B	-1.50	-0.154		-0.154		-0.154		-0.154	
11M	-1.74	-0.190	-0.190		-0.190			-0.190	
12M	-1.23	-0.274	-0.274		-0.274			-0.274	
13M	-0.47	-0.099			-0.099			-0.099	
14M	-0.87	-0.502	-0.502		-0.502			-0.502	
15M	-1.49	-0.862		-0.862	-0.862			-0.862	
16M	-3.70	-0.597	-0.597		-0.597			-0.597	
17M	0.00	0.000				0.000			0.000
18M	-1.11	-0.248		-0.248	-0.248			-0.248	
21M	-0.97	-0.175				-0.175			-0.175
22M	-1.48	-0.557				-0.557			-0.557
24M	0.00	0.015				0.015			0.015
25M	0.31	0.036			0.036				0.036

d. Vigor Scores -- POMS Studies

Study	Z	ES	ES-m	ES-f	ES-ya	ES-ma	ES-ea	ES-sur	ES-exp
1M-M	0.36	0.135	0.135		0.135				0.135
1M-F	1.63	0.517		0.517	0.517				0.517
3M	1.71	0.677				0.677			0.677
7M	-0.54	-0.119		-0.119	-0.119				-0.119
9M-M	3.70	0.904	0.904			0.904		0.904	

(table continues)

(Table 6.3, continued)

Study	Z	ES	ES-m	ES-f	ES-ya	ES-ma	ES-ea	ES-sur	ES-exp
9M-F	3.70	0.634		0.634		0.634		0.634	
10M-A	3.70	0.696		0.696		0.696		0.696	
10M-B	3.70	0.404		0.404		0.404		0.404	
11M	-3.08	-0.333	-0.333		-0.333			-0.333	
12M	1.64	0.363	0.363		0.363			0.363	
13M	1.40	0.303			0.303			0.303	
14M	1.05	0.612	0.612		0.612			0.612	
15M	1.51	0.874		0.874	0.874			0.874	
16M	3.70	0.910	0.910		0.910			0.910	
17M	0.00	0.000				0.000			0.000
18M	1.96	0.438		0.438	0.438			0.438	
21M	0.60	0.107				0.107			0.107
22M	0.93	0.340				0.340			0.340
24M	0.48	0.108				0.108			0.108
25M	3.40	0.412			0.412				0.412

e. Fatigue Scores -- POMS Studies

Study	Z	ES	ES-m	ES-f	ES-ya	ES-ma	ES-ea	ES-sur	ES-exp
1M-M	0.44	0.164	0.164		0.164				0.164
1M-F	-1.33	-0.422		-0.422	-0.422				-0.422
3M	-2.07	-0.833				-0.833			-0.833
7M	0.00	-0.016		-0.016	-0.016				-0.016
9M-M	-3.70	-0.489	-0.489			-0.489		-0.489	
9M-F	-3.70	-0.407		-0.407		-0.407		-0.407	
10M-A	1.03	0.130	0.130			0.130		0.130	
10M-B	-0.71	-0.072		-0.072		-0.072		-0.072	
11M	-3.70	-0.483	-0.483		-0.483			-0.483	
12M	-1.78	-0.400	-0.400		-0.400			-0.400	
13M	-0.19	-0.040			-0.040			-0.040	
14M	-0.56	-0.319	-0.319		-0.319			-0.319	
15M	-0.93	-0.514		-0.514	-0.514			-0.514	
16M	-3.70	-0.565	-0.565		-0.565			-0.565	
17M	0.00	0.000				0.000			0.000
18M	-0.64	-0.142		-0.142	-0.142			-0.142	
21M	-1.26	-0.227				-0.227			-0.227
22M	-1.75	-0.660				-0.660			-0.660
24M	-0.59	-0.100				-0.100			-0.100
25M	-0.24	-0.028			-0.028				-0.028

(table continues)

(Table 6.3, continued)

Study	Z	ES	ES-m	ES-f	ES-ya	ES-ma	ES-ea	ES-sur	ES-exp
			f. Confusion Scores -- POMS Studies						
1M-M	-0.16	-0.060	-0.060		-0.060				-0.060
1M-F	-1.42	-0.454		-0.454	-0.454				-0.454
3M	0.00	0.000				0.000			0.000
7M	-0.86	-0.190		-0.190	-0.190				-0.190
9M-M	-3.70	-0.824	-0.824			-0.824		-0.824	
9M-F	-3.70	-0.699		-0.699		-0.699		-0.699	
10M-A	-0.53	-0.067		-0.067		-0.067		-0.067	
10M-B	-1.37	-0.140		-0.140		-0.140		-0.140	
11M	-3.70	-0.768	-0.768		-0.768			-0.768	
12M	-2.60	-0.591	-0.591		-0.591			-0.591	
13M	-1.88	-0.405			-0.405			-0.405	
14M	-1.21	-0.706	-0.706		-0.706			-0.706	
15M	-1.76	-1.029		-1.029	-1.029			-1.029	
16M	-3.70	-0.532	-0.532		-0.532			-0.532	
17M	0.00	0.000				0.000			0.000
18M	-0.88	-0.195		-0.195	-0.195			-0.195	
21M	-1.96	-0.353				-0.353			-0.353
22M	-2.29	-0.869				-0.869			-0.869
24M	0.33	0.073				0.073			0.073
25M	-1.98	-0.229			-0.229				-0.229

*See text for definitions of column heads.

Table 6.4. Z scores and effect sizes as calculated for each study.*

Study	Z	ES	ES-m	ES-f	ES-ya	ES-ma	ES-ea	ES-sur	ES-exp
					a. Anxiety Scores -- MAACL Studies				
4M	-1.68	-1.652				-1.652			-1.652
5M	-3.11	-1.157	-1.157			-1.157			-1.157
6M-M	-1.13	-0.374	-0.374		-0.374				-0.374
6M-F	-3.11	-1.060		-1.060	-1.060				-1.060
8M	-1.11	-1.678				-1.678		-1.678	
19M	-1.75	-0.582					-0.582		-0.582
20M	-3.70	-0.556		-0.556		-0.556		-0.556	
23M	0.00	0.000		0.000		0.000			0.000
26M-M	-1.12	-0.645	-0.645			-0.645			-0.645
26M-F	-3.30	-2.219		-2.219		-2.219			-2.219
					b. Depression Scores -- MAACL Studies				
4M	-2.30	-2.534				-2.534			-2.534
5M	-2.17	-0.792	-0.792			-0.792			-0.792
6M-M	-0.79	-0.263	-0.263		-0.263				-0.263
6M-F	-2.98	-1.016		-1.016	-1.016				-1.016
8M	-1.42	-2.273				-2.273		-2.273	
23M	0.00	0.000		0.000		0.000			0.000
26M-M	-0.53	-0.293	-0.293			-0.293			-0.293
26M-F	-2.83	-1.813		-1.813		-1.813			-1.813
					c. Hostility Scores -- MAACL Studies				
4M	-1.14	-1.071				-1.071			-1.071
8M	-0.60	-0.793				-0.793		-0.793	
23M	0.00	0.000		0.000		0.000			0.000

*See text for definitions of column heads.

4. ES-m: Effect size for male subjects (if any) in that study.
5. ES-f: Effect size for female subjects (if any) in that study. No entry for male or female subjects indicates that sex of subjects was not given, or results were given for a mixed male/female group, with no gender breakdown.
6. ES-ya: Effect size for young adult (<30) subjects, if any.
7. ES-ma: Effect size for middle-aged (>30) adults, if any.
8. ES-ea: Effect size for elderly (>60) adults, if any.
9. ES-sur: Effect size for studies based on data from surveys or pre-experimental designs.
10. ES-exp: Effect size for studies based on data from true or quasi-experimental designs.

Results by Group

Results of the meta-analysis of the mood group are summarized in Tables 6.5, based on the data given in Tables 6.3 and 6.4.

Column headings for Table 6.5 are as follows:

1. Measure: The standard scales on the POMS and MAACL, respectively. N = the number of studies reporting data for each scale.
2. Zst: The standard normal deviate score for all of the reports combined.
3. Mn-ES: Mean effect size (ES) and standard error for all reports combined. Negative ES = decrease in mean ES.
4. ES-m: Mean ES and standard error for all male subjects combined.
5. ES-f: Mean ES and standard error for all female subjects combined.
6. ES-ya: Mean ES and standard error for all young adult (<30) groups combined.
7. ES-ma: Mean ES and standard error for all middle-aged (>30) adult groups combined.
8. ES-ea: Mean ES and standard error for all elderly (>60) groups combined.

Table 6.5. Z scores, mean effect sizes (first row) and standard
errors (second row) for each scale.*

Measure Zst	Mn-ES	ES-m ES-f	ES-ya ES-ma ES-ea	ES-sur ES-exp

a. POMS Studies

Tension				
N = 20 -6.666	-0.322	-0.433 -0.254	-0.323 -0.322	-0.312 -0.335
p<.00001	0.060	0.038 0.093	0.063 0.113	0.059 0.117
Anger				
N = 21 -2.856	-0.182	-0.286 -0.119	-0.277 0.020 -0.950	-0.197 -0.163
p<.0021	0.068	0.143 0.095	0.081 0.051 --	0.089 0.113
Depression				
N = 20 -5.501	-0.284	-0.343 -0.275	-0.303 -0.260	-0.314 -0.247
p<.00001	0.068	0.073 0.134	0.090 0.111	0.080 0.121
Vigor				
N = 20 7.055	0.399	0.432 0.492	0.374 0.430	0.528 0.242
p<.00001	0.077	0.197 0.119	0.114 0.105	0.109 0.087
Fatigue				
N = 20 -5.675	-0.271	-0.349 -0.206	-0.251 -0.295	-0.300 -0.236
p<.00001	0.062	0.108 0.092	0.075 0.108	0.070 0.112
Confusion				
N = 20 -7.462	-0.402	-0.580 -0.396	-0.469 -0.320	-0.541 -0.231
p<.00001	0.075	0.113 0.134	0.088 0.127	0.093 0.099

b. MAACL Studies

Anxiety				
N = 10 -6.328	-0.988	-0.720 -0.955	-0.715 -1.124 -0.582	-1.110 -0.958
p<.00001	0.218	0.229 0.471	0.345 0.292 --	0.560 0.254
Depression				
N = 8 -4.603	-1.120	-0.447 -0.940	-0.635 -1.282	-2.273 -0.956
p<.0001	0.343	0.172 0.524	0.375 0.435	-- 0.348
Hostility				
N = 3 1.005				
N.S.				

*See text for definitions of column heads.

9.   ES-sur: Mean ES and standard error for all reports based on data from surveys or pre-experimental designs.

10. ES-exp: Mean ES and standard error for all reports based on data from true or quasi-experimental designs.

In all cases, a negative mean ES indicates that the experimental group showed a decrease from pre- to posttest, or scored lower than control subjects or norm groups, or both.

The formula for calculation of Z_{st} is

$$Z_{st} = \frac{\text{sum } Z_{1-N}}{\text{square root of N}}$$

This formula, sometimes called adding Zs, is described by Rosenthal (1978) and by Cooper (1989). Calculations for all other values in Table 6.5 are straightforward and in the usual manner.

Statistical significance of the results was evaluated by two methods. First, the combined Z scores, obtained by adding Zs, were interpreted in the usual way, that is, a Z score of 1.645 was required for the overall effect on any one scale to reach significance at $p<.05$ (one-tailed test) within the standard normal deviate.

Based on a wealth of previous research, we predicted a priori that (1) all scores on the POMS would show a decrease, except vigor which would show an increase, and (2) all scores on the MAACL would show a decrease. Planned comparisons were then made in those cases where the Z score did reach statistical significance. Following the model used by Smith (1980), Smith, Glass, and Miller (1980), and Landman and Dawes (1982), it was concluded that mean ESs were shown to differ reliably from one another only if the difference between them was more than two standard errors, using the greater of the two standard errors. Thus, differences in the planned comparisons were judged to be statistically significant only when the mean of the experimental group exceeded 97.5% of the values in the control or pretest observation. This is a relatively simple, but conservative, criterion that is probably well recommended whenever the number of planned comparisons becomes great enough that the likelihood of Type I error may be excessive.

POMS

1. Main effects. As shown in Table 6.5a, all six scales of the POMS showed significant overall effects, with the Z scores ranging from 2.856 (anger) to 7.462 (confusion). Thus, all scales changed at $p<.01$ or better. Five of the six scales showed a decrease, whereas the vigor scale showed an increase, highly consistent with much previous research with the POMS.

2. Male-female differences. Both male and female groups showed significant changes in tension, depression, vigor, fatigue, and confusion but no significant change in anger scores.

3. Age differences. Young adults showed reliable decreases on the usual five scales, and a significant increase in vigor scores. Middle-aged groups showed significant decreases in tension, depression, fatigue and confusion, plus a significant increase in vigor scores. The single elderly group reported in this set apparently showed the largest decrease in anger scores, although this may not be reliable.

4. Survey versus experiment differences. Both the survey and the experiment reports in this grouping showed significant decreases in tension, depression, fatigue and confusion scores, plus a significant increase in vigor scores. The survey studies showed significant changes in anger scores, but not the experiment studies.

5. Differences by type of effect size calculation. Type of ES ratings (given in Table 6.2) indicated no reliable differences between mean effect sizes based on (1) the full formula, (2) the briefer Glass formula, (3) *t*, *F*, or chi-square statistics, or (4) those using norm data as controls.

6. Differences by type of exercise. Three of the studies in the present group reported using fitness exercises other than run/jog. These were Berger and Owen (1983) who used swimming, Blumenthal, Schocken, Needels, and Hindle (1982) who used a stationary bike, and Johnson et al. (1985) who used cycling. In general, the results of these three studies were not different in any reliable manner from the remainder of the group. The only possible exception was the vigor score in the Johnson et al. study which was reported to decrease after training, notably because reported decreases in this scale are somewhat unusual.

MAACL

1. Main effects. As shown in Table 6.5b, two of the three scales on the MAACL (anxiety and depression) showed a significant overall decrease, with Z scores of 6.328 and 4.603, respectively, whereas the third (hostility) was not significant, with Z = 1.005. All following comments are therefore be limited to the anxiety and depression scales.

2. Male-female differences. Male groups showed reliable decreases in both anxiety and depression scores. Females showed an anxiety score decrease, but the decrease in depression scores was not reliable.

3. Age differences. Both young and middle-aged adults showed reliable decreases in anxiety and depression scores, with the middle-aged group showing consistently larger decreases, although not significantly larger than the young adults.

4. Survey versus experiment differences. Both survey and experiment reports showed significant decreases in both anxiety and depression scores; however, the decrease in depression scores in the survey reports was reliably larger than that in the experiment reports.

5. Differences by type of effect size calculation. There were no consistent differences between reports based on differences in method of calculating effect sizes.

6. Differences by type of exercise. As shown in Table 6.2b, all of the studies in this group used run/jog as the fitness exercise, hence no comparisons across types of exercise were possible.

POMS and MAACL Compared

On the basis of the foregoing analyses, it should be possible to make some comparative statements about the relative findings with the POMS versus the MAACL. Both scales showed consistently significant decreases in tension/anxiety scores and depression scores. In addition, both scales showed the smallest change in anger/hostility scores, with the latter being not significant on the MAACL. To this extent, the overall results appear to be similar with either instrument.

On the other hand, the effect sizes resulting from the MAACL studies are consistently and reliably larger than those derived from the POMS. Although the cause of this difference is not certain to us, it is likely that the previously mentioned proclivity for MAACL scores to be influenced by response sets may be an important factor. Therefore the POMS may be the less set-influenced than the MAACL, perhaps because of differences in the question format, that is, it is easier to be influenced by transients such as set in choosing any adjectives to check *at all* on the MAACL, as opposed to the decision process involved in rating all adjectives 0-4 on the POMS.

The POMS offers the further advantage that it includes the vigor scale, which has been shown to *increase* in many exercise-related studies.

General Findings

Taken as a single set, the results of the meta-analysis of the mood studies can be summarized as follows:

1. Both the POMS and the MAACL studies indicate significant overall effects on mood, most notably a decrease in tension/anxiety and depression (POMS and MAACL), a decrease in fatigue and confusion (POMS), plus an increase in vigor (POMS).

2. Both male and female groups show these changes on both instruments, except that the decrease in female MAACL depression scores was not significant.

3. Young adults and middle-aged adults both showed all of the foregoing changes. Too few elderly groups were reported to draw any conclusions about this age group.

4. Comparison of the survey-versus-experiment reports, intended as an index of the rigor of designs, showed that one should probably discount changes in the anger scores on the POMS.

5. There was no evidence that the results were influenced by method of calculating effect sizes. There were no indications of differences in effects across fitness exercises, although there were minimal opportunities for such comparisons.

6. The overall magnitude of effect sizes suggested that the POMS may be less susceptible to test-taking attitude or response sets than the MAACL.

7. None of the studies in this total set mentioned follow-up testing at some later date after completion of fitness training. Hence these studies should be interpreted as measuring immediate or short-term effects, which means that there are no data on long-term effects on mood at this time.

Interpretation of Findings

Although we wish to postpone a theoretical interpretation of the apparent effects of aerobic fitness training on mood, some general interpretations are in order at this point. First, it has been well demonstrated that aerobic fitness training produces some positive change in mood, as reflected on both the POMS and the MAACL, although there are some differences attributable to sex and age. Therefore some of the warranted conclusions should be worded cautiously, but this does not alter the fact that change *does* occur, at least on a short-term basis. Moods are defined as transient feeling states, and so the lack of long-term data may constitute a partly unsolvable problem.

The primary mood changes were decreases in tension/anxiety, depression, fatigue and confusion, plus an increase in vigor. The decreases in POMS depression scores were significantly less than the decreases seen in the depression group as described in chapter 7.

The results should also be interpreted cautiously in light of likely effects of test-taking attitude or response set on the results. The evidence does seem to suggest that the MAACL may be more susceptible to such response sets, and this should be kept in mind when drawing conclusions based on data from this instrument.

A troublesome number of authors omitted age and/or gender data about their subjects, and several reports were therefore not included in the planned comparisons related to age or gender. Similarly, only one study used elderly subjects, hence our planned age comparisons were necessarily restricted.

Investigators in this area routinely omit reference to problems with response sets, with one notable exception. Berger and Owen (1983) included the Lie scale of the Eysenck Personality Inventory (Eysenck & Eysenck, 1963) as an independent measure of social desirability, and they were able to show that this did not differ across groups. Such recognition of an existing problem is strongly encouraged in future work, even though it does not constitute a full solution to the larger problem of biased results due to response sets.

Finally, although one might normally turn at this point to a consideration of the mechanisms whereby fitness training produces positive mood effects, we postpone discussion of theory to chapter 10, after first reviewing the research in other related areas. This is particularly true of research on the effects of fitness training on anxiety and depression. Data presented in this chapter clearly indicate that fitness training has its greatest positive effects on reducing anxiety and depression (and increasing vigor) *in groups of normal subjects*. In chapter 7 we examine the effects of fitness training as a potential *therapeutic* device in dealing with depression or anxiety, clearly a body of research that is highly relevant to the overall question of mechanisms for fitness training effects on mood.

Summary

Our meta-analysis of studies on the effects of aerobic fitness training on mood states can be summarized as follows:

1. Mood states were defined as transient feelings or affective states, in contrast to more enduring characteristics such as self-concept or personality traits.

2. The two standardized tests used to measure moods, the POMS and MAACL, were described. Some of the prominent features and possible problems were outlined.

3. The total set of mood studies (both the POMS and the MAACL groups) were described, including groups, number of males versus females, mean age, experimental design, type of effect size, fitness exercise, and measure of fitness.

4. The results of the meta-analyses of both groups were presented, and the rationale for statistical comparisons explained, including the method of adding Zs, and planned comparisons between effect sizes of subgroupings.

5. Results for both the POMS and the MAACL were described, including main effects, sex differences, age differences, and differences by type of experimental design, type of effect size, and type of fitness exercise.

6. Both the POMS and the MAACL showed significant decreases in tension/anxiety and depression scores, while vigor scores (on the POMS) increased. fatigue and confusion scores (POMS) also decreased significantly. Data derived from MAACL studies appeared to be more susceptible to response set biases.

7. The decreases in POMS depression scores were significantly less than the decrease in depression scores seen in the depression group in chapter 7.

8. Other differences as a result of sex or age were outlined. The more rigorous studies using the POMS failed to find significant changes in anger scores. There were no effects based on type of ES calculation or type of fitness exercise.

9. Several tentative interpretations were suggested, but postponed for more detailed consideration in chapter 10, so that all of the data could be considered more fully.

SEVEN

DEPRESSION AND ANXIETY

This chapter reviews studies that measure changes in depression and/or anxiety as a result of aerobic fitness training. The interest in depression and anxiety results from the hope that aerobic fitness training has a positive therapeutic effect.

Aerobic fitness programs (primarily running/jogging, dance, swimming, or walking) have come to be frequent prescriptions for treating depression. Consequently, some of the studies in this group include subjects with various levels of reported symptomatic difficulty, although not necessarily patients in a treatment program. Clearly, the preferred goal in such studies is to establish that fitness training has had a relatively lasting therapeutic effect, rather than some mood change for one brief moment. As such, the definition of depression and/or anxiety is more trait than state, even though many writers continue to find it useful to describe depression as a "mood disorder."

Nevertheless, the distinction between the depression and anxiety studies in this chapter, and the mood studies reviewed in chapter 6, is imperfect at best. Although the mood studies are generally addressed toward more global measures of mood change (especially those in which the POMS was used. since this scale includes six different measures of mood), the depression and anxiety studies are more narrowly defined or unidimensional. For example, scales designed to measure depression or anxiety generally yield one score of depression, or one score of anxiety, as opposed to a profile of several scores over several dimensions.

There is, however, at least one exception, namely, the State-Trait Anxiety Inventory, a questionnaire that yields two measures of anxiety: state anxiety and trait anxiety. Anxiety as a state is intended to focus on the individual's present feelings, and thus seems to overlap with our use of the concept of mood as a relatively transient feeling. Anxiety as a trait, however, is a more enduring characteristic and therefore should probably not be classed as a mood in the transient sense. Examples might include anxiety as a more long-term trait in cases of anxiety neurosis or in Type A behavior pattern, the heart disease prone personality syndrome.

Thus, our distinction between mood studies and studies of depression and anxiety is partly conceptual, but also partly methodological, and partly to clarify the presentation of our findings in an area where the definition of key terms is not always consistent.

Measures of Depression

Five standardized tests have been used in studies of depression: (1) the Beck Depression Inventory (DI), (2) the Center for Epidemiological Studies Depression Scale (CES-D Scale), (3) the Lubin Depression Adjective Check Lists (Lubin DACL), (4) the Symptom Check List--90 (SCL--90), and (5) the Zung Self-Rating Depression Scale (Zung SDS).

Beck DI
The Beck DI was developed by Aaron Beck in 1967, a psychiatrist, and is frequently employed in a variety of studies on depression. The DI consists of 21 clusters of statements. Each cluster consists of four to six statements rank-ordered to assess one behavior or symptom aspect of depression, such as sadness, pessimism, sense of failure, dissatisfaction, guilt, and so on, and scored from 0 to 3 for degree of severity. Scores on the DI can thus range from 0 to 63, although normal subjects reportedly average 5 to 10, and moderately to severely depressed subjects average approximately 25 to 30 (Beck, 1967; p. 196). Although the instructions specify that the statements be read individually to subjects, the DI can be given in pencil-and-paper format. In this latter form, the inventory has the advantage that it can be taken in 5 to 10 minutes by most subjects. Subjects are instructed to respond in terms of how they feel "today, that is, right now."

Center for Epidemiological Studies Depression Scale
Development of the CES-D Scale was summarized by Lenore Radloff (1977). The scale consists of 20 items to

which subjects are instructed to respond on a four-step scale from "rarely" to "all the time" in the past week. The items were drawn from a pool of items derived from five previously validated depression scales, including the Beck DI and the Zung SDS. Data on reliability, validity, factor structure and correlations with other scales are given by Radloff. The CES-D Scale should therefore prove to be at least as useful and/or as limited as other existing scales.

Lubin Depression Adjective Check Lists

The Lubin DACL were introduced by Bernard Lubin (1965, 1981), and, like the Beck Inventory, have shown broad use by a large number of investigators in a variety of studies on depression. There are seven forms of the DACL, each of which consists of 32 or 34 adjectives related to depression or elation. Subjects are instructed to check those words that describe "how you feel now--today." The DACL is thus open-ended with regard to the number of adjectives a subject may check. Normative data given by Lubin (1981, pp. 6-7) indicate that normal subjects may give average scores of 7 to 8, whereas depressed patients average 13 to 18. Goodstein (1972a) in a review of the DACL, was generally positive in tone, however, McNair (1972), in a related review, was more critical, citing the finding that the DACL appears to measure affective states beyond depression, a problem that may be common to all questionnaire measures of depression. The DACL thus appears to be no better or worse than the DI (or any other questionnaire) in terms of apparent advantages or disadvantages.

Symptom Check List -- 90

The SCL-90 was developed by Derogatis and colleagues (Derogatis, Lipman, & Covi, 1973; Derogatis, Rickels, & Rock, 1976). It consists of a 90-symptom check list over a diverse array of problem areas. Subjects are asked to rate each symptom from 0 to 4 (from "not at all" to "extremely") to indicate how much discomfort they have experienced within the last week for each symptom. The scale provides a total of nine different factor scores, but only one of these is depression, which consists of 13 items of the total of 90. It is possible to give the depression scale individually. Pauker (1985) was generally positive in describing the SCL-90, whereas Payne (1985) was more critical, indicating that the SCL-90 may measure no more than a general factor of complaining about symptoms. Although the test-retest reliability data appear to be within normally acceptable limits, we question whether investigators would be wise to stake an entire research program on subjects' responses to 13 items.

Zung Self-Rating Depression Scale

The Zung SDS was developed by the psychiatrist, William Zung (1965, 1969). The SDS consists of 20 items, which are scored from 1 to 4 (from "a little of the time" to "most of the time") in contrast to the "now" or "in the past week" emphasis of the three foregoing inventories. Half of the items reflect depressive feeling, and the other half reflect more positive feeling and are scored in the opposite direction. Raw scores may range from 20 to 80; however, Zung reports using an SDS "index," which is simply the raw score divided by 80 (the maximum possible score). Goodstein (1972b) points out that Zung has not reported reliability data, that scores are "easily faked," and he suggests that the DACL may therefore be more useful than the SDS, a point to which we return below.

Measures of Anxiety

Two standardized tests have been used in studies of anxiety: (1) the Manifest Anxiety Scale (MAS), and (2) the State-Trait Anxiety Inventory (STAI).

Taylor Manifest Anxiety Scale

The MAS was initially reported by Janet Taylor (1951, 1953). The scale consists of 50 true-false items taken from the 500-item pool of the Minnesota Multiphasic Personality Inventory (MMPI). It is intended to be a measure of trait anxiety, a more enduring characteristic than state anxiety. The MAS was shown by Taylor to predict strength of eyelid conditioning, which she interpreted as an index of drive or motivation. Because the MAS is imbedded within the MMPI, as well as other features, the MAS has been used by many investigators since Taylor's first report.   It can be given separately, or as a part of the full MMPI.

Spielberger State-Trait Anxiety Inventory

The STAI was developed by Charles Spielberger and colleagues (Spielberger, 1983; Spielberger, Gorsuch, & Lushene, 1970).   The STAI consists of two 20-item scales, one to measure state anxiety, and one to measure trait anxiety.   Instructions on the state scale direct subjects to respond how they feel "right now," whereas the instructions in the trait scale direct subjects to respond in terms of how they feel "generally."   Items in both scales consist of statements that are answered from 1 to 4, indicating "not at all" to "very much so" on the state scale, and those on the trait scale are answered "almost never" to "almost always."   The total STAI is therefore somewhat briefer than the MAS.   At the present time, the STAI is a widely used measure of anxiety, and both Dreger (1978) and Katkin (1978) were generally positive in their overall assessment of the STAI as a measure of anxiety, although some limitations were noted.

Independent Variables

Fifteen studies were identified that met all selection criteria and constitute the depression group.   The 15 studies, including identification number (alphabetical by first author), authors, year of publication, and depression scale used are given in Table 7.1a.   Similarly, 22 studies that qualified constitute the anxiety group, and the identifying information on these studies is given in Table 7.1b.   Four studies (Blumenthal, Emery, Madden, George, Coleman, Riddle, McKee, Reasoner, & Williams, 1989; Hannaford, Harrell, & Cox, 1988; Hayden & Allen, 1984; Morgan & Pollock, 1977) qualified for both the depression and anxiety groups because the authors used measures of depression and anxiety as listed.   In addition, nine of the studies listed in Table 7.1 were included in the mood group (see Table 6.1), namely, Blumenthal, Williams, et al. (1982), Johnson et al. (1985), Kowal et al. (1978), Morgan and Pollock (1977), Morgan et al. (1987, 1988), Perri and Templer (1984-85), Steptoe et al. (1989), and Williams and Getty

Table 7.1. Studies, showing identification number, authors,
year of publication, and scale used.

ID	Authors	Year	Scale

a. Depression Group

ID	Authors	Year	Scale
1D	Blumenthal et al.	1989	CES-D
2D	Brown, Ramirez, and Taub	1978	Zung
3D	Doyne, Ossip-Klein, Bowman, Osborn, McDougall-Wilson, and Neimeyer	1987	Beck & Lubin
4D	Hannaford et al.	1988	Zung
5D	Hayden and Allen	1984	Beck
6D	Jasnoski and Holmes	1981	Zung
7D	Klein, Greist, Gurman, Neimeyer, Lesser, Bushnell, and Smith	1985	SCL-90
8D	McCann and Holmes	1984	Beck
9D	Morgan and Costill	1972	Lubin
10D	Morgan and Pollock	1977	Lubin
11D	Morgan, Roberts, Brand, and Feinerman	1970	Zung
12D	Parent and Whall	1984	Beck
13D	Perri and Templer	1984-85	Zung
14D	Rape	1987	Beck
15D	Williams and Getty	1986	Zung

b. Anxiety Group

ID	Authors	Year	Scale
1A	Abadie	1988	STAI-Trait
2A	Blumenthal et al.	1989	STAI

(table continues)

(Table 7.1, continued)

ID	Authors	Year	Scale
3A	Blumenthal, Williams, et al.	1982	STAI
4A	Goldwater and Collis	1985	MAS
5A	Hammer and Wilmore	1973	MAS
6A	Hannaford et al.	1988	STAI-State
7A	Hayden and Allen	1984	STAI
8A	Johnson et al.	1985	STAI
9A	Kowal et al.	1978	STAI
10A	Leste and Rust	1984	STAI-State
11A	Long and Haney	1988	STAI-Trait
12A	Maloney, Cheney, Spring, and Kanusky	1986	STAI-Trait
13A	McGlynn, Franklin, Lauro, and McGlynn	1983	STAI
14A	Morgan et al.	1988	STAI
15A	Morgan et al.	1987	STAI
16A	Morgan and Pollock	1977	STAI
17A	Netz, Tenenbaum, and Sagiv	1988	STAI-Trait
18A	Nouri and Beer	1989	STAI-Trait
19A	Pauly, Palmer, Wright, and Pfeiffer	1982	STAI-Trait
20A	Shephard and Cox	1980	MAS
21A	Sinyor, Schwartz, Peronnet, Brisson, and Seraganian	1983	STAI
22A	Steptoe et al.	1989	STAI-Trait

(1986), in each case because of the use of two or more qualifying questionnaires as dependent variables.

Specific design characteristics of the studies in the depression group and in the anxiety group are given in Table 7.2. Following the same format used in chapter 6, the table gives: identification number, number of groups, number of subjects per group, number of male and female subjects, mean age, experimental design and type of effect size, fitness exercise, and measure(s) of fitness. There were two independent samples in the Brown et al. (1978) report, hence they are treated as two studies in the meta-analysis. Gaps in the gender and age columns indicate information that was not reported by the authors, although in several instances it was still possible to estimate the approximate age of subjects, as can be seen in both Tables 7.3 and 7.4. The rating systems for experimental design and type of effect size are described in detail in chapter 6.

Results by Study

Z scores and effect sizes for each study in the depression group and in the anxiety group are summarized in Table 7.3 (a and b, respectively). The column headings in Table 7.3 are the same as those used in chapter 6. The dependent variable for each study in Table 7.3a was the effect size calculated from a single depression score, regardless of instrument, whereas in Table 7.3b, the results for three anxiety scores are summarized individually: the state and trait scores of the STAI, plus the anxiety score from the MAS. As explained in chapters 5 and 6, the information about each individual study in Tables 7.1 to 7.3 is given primarily to promote the replicability of our analysis.

Depression and Anxiety Groups -- Results by Group

Results of the meta-analyses of the Depression and anxiety groups are summarized in Table 7.4, based exclusively on the data given in Table 7.3. All column headings in Table 7.4 are the same as those used in chapter 6.

Table 7.2. Independent Variables.

Study	No. of Groups	Ne	Nc	Nm	Nf	Age	Design/ES-type	Fitness Exercise	Measure of Fitness
							a. Depression Group		
1D-M	2m	17	16	33	--	66.7	4/3	bike, jog	VO2max
1D-F	2f	16	18	--	34	66.7	4/3	bike, jog	VO2max
*2D-A	1	26	54	--	--	20?	10/1	jog 5x/wk	HR, 12-min run
*2D-B	1	65	383	--	--	20?	10/1	jog 3x/wk	HR, 12-min run
*3D	2	13	13	--	26	29	4/1	walk/run	treadmill
*4D	2	9	9	18	--	40?	4/3	run	1.5 mi run
5D	2	34	30	--	--	18.7	10/3	run	aer. pts.
6D	1	103	--	--	103	20.3	2/3	run+	12-min run
*7D	1	15	--	--	--	30?	4/4	run	program completion
*8D	2	15	14	--	29	20?	4/3	run+	12-min run
9D	1	9	--	9	--	32	1/4	marathon	running history
10D	1	27	--	27	--	24.8	1/4	elite runners	running history
11D	2	23	16	39	--	40?	10/1	jog	HR, %BF, VO2max
12D	1	30	--	--	--	60?	3/3	running history	running history
13D	2	23	19	14	28	65.4	10/1	walk/jog	compulsory class
14D	2	21	21	42	--	20?	3/2	running history	running history
*15D	2	24	9	--	--	20?	10/1	jog/dance	class completion

(table continues)

(Table 7.2. continued)

Study	No. of Groups	Ne	Nc	Nm	Nf	Age	Design/ ES-type	Fitness Exercise	Measure of Fitness
				b. Anxiety Group					
1A	1	32	--	8	24	68.2	1/3	walk	VO2max
2A-M	2m	17	16	33	--	66.7	4/3	bike, jog	VO2max
2A-F	2f	16	18	--	34	66.7	4/3	bike, jog	VO2max
3A	2	16	16	10	22	45.1	10/3	walk/jog	BP, HR, Wt
4A	2	14	18	32	--	22?	10/2	run+	step test
5A	2	9	9	18	--	30?	10/2	jog	VO2max
6A	2	9	9	18	--	40?	4/3	run	1.5-mi run
7A	2	34	30	--	--	18.7	10/3	run	aer. pts.
8A	1	6	--	6	--	21	2/4	cycling	%BF, VO2max
9A	1	85	--	85	--	20?	2/4	basic training	%BF, VO2max
10A	2	23	38	--	--	19.9	10/1	dance	program completion
11A	2	25	25	--	50	39.8	4/1	jog	program completion
12A-M	1m	15	--	15	--	34.0	1/2	run	step test, 2-mi run
12A-F	1f	28	--	--	28	29.6	1/2	run	step test, 2-mi run
13A	2	15	15	--	--	20?	10/1	walk/jog	step test
14A	1	14	--	14	--	26.4	1/4	running history	running history
15A	1	15	--	--	15	27.2	1/4	running history	running history
16A	1	27	--	27	--	24.8	1/4	elite runners	VO2max

(table continues)

(Table 7.2, continued)

Study	No. of Groups	Ne	Nc	Nm	Nf	Age	Design/ ES-type	Fitness Exercise	Measure of Fitness
17A-M	1m	11	--	11	--	60.4	2/2	walk/jog	treadmill
17A-F	1f	13	--	--	13	55.8	2/2	walk/jog	treadmill
18A	2	20	25	45	--	37	1/3	running history	running history
19A	1	73	--	--	--	36	2/3	run/bike	%BF, HR, VO2max
20A	2	153	142	133	162	34.5	10/3	jog	%BF, LBM, VO2max
21A	2	15	15	30	--	26	3/3	run	HR, aer. pts., VO2max
22A	2	17	16	5	28	37.0	10/1	walk/run	bike ergometer

Note: Ne and Nc = number of subjects in the experimental and control groups; Nm and Nf = number of male and female subjects; Age = mean for the total group; HR = heart rate, %BF = percent body fat. Asterisk indicates studies with depressed subjects.

Table 7.3. Z scores and effect sizes as calculated for each study.

Study	Z	Mn-ES	ES-m	ES-f	ES-ya	ES-ma	ES-ea	ES-sur	ES-exp
a. Depression Group									
1D-M	-2.46	-1.465	-1.465				-1.465		-1.465
1D-F	0.00	0.000		0.000			0.000		0.000
2D-A	-4.00	-2.415			-2.415				-2.415
2D-B	-4.00	-1.158			-1.158				-1.158
3D	-2.71	-1.339		-1.339	-1.339				-1.339
4D	-1.43	-0.754	-0.754			-0.754			-0.754
5D	-3.70	-1.070			-1.070				-1.070
6D	0.00	0.000		0.000	0.000			0.000	
7D	-4.00	-1.018				-1.018			-1.018
8D	-2.87	-1.287		-1.287	-1.287				-1.287
9D	-2.91	-1.808	-1.808			-1.808		-1.808	
10D	-4.00	-1.988	-1.988		-1.988			-1.988	
11D	1.50	0.397	0.397			0.397			0.397
12D	-3.11	-0.923					-0.923	-0.923	
13D	-1.43	-0.470					-0.470		-0.470
14D	-2.65	-0.939	-0.939		-0.939			-0.939	
15D	-0.56	-0.206			-0.206				-0.206

b. Anxiety Group

A. State Scores

Study	Z	Mn-ES	ES-m	ES-f	ES-ya	ES-ma	ES-ea	ES-sur	ES-exp
2A-M	0.00	0.000	0.000			0.000			0.000
2A-F	0.00	0.000		0.000		0.000			0.000
3A	-1.87	-0.776				-0.776			-0.776
6A	-0.83	-0.413	-0.413			-0.413			-0.413
7A	-2.55	-0.599			-0.599				-0.599
8A	0.00	0.000	0.000		0.000			0.000	
9A	-1.74	-0.391	-0.391		-0.391			-0.391	
10A	-4.00	-0.993		-0.993	-0.993				-0.993
13A	-0.64	-0.246			-0.246				-0.246
14A	0.00	0.006	0.006		0.006			0.006	
15A	0.00	0.069		0.069	0.069			0.069	
16A	-0.72	-0.287	-0.287		-0.287			-0.287	
21A	0.00	0.000	0.000		0.000			0.000	

B. Trait Scores

Study	Z	Mn-ES	ES-m	ES-f	ES-ya	ES-ma	ES-ea	ES-sur	ES-exp
1A	0.00	0.011					0.011	0.011	
2A-M	-1.48	-0.324	-0.324				-0.324		-0.324

(table continues)

(Table 7.3, continued)

Study	Z	Mn-ES	ES-m	ES-f	ES-ya	ES-ma	ES-ea	ES-sur	ES-exp
2A-F	0.00	0.000		0.000			0.000		0.000
3A	-2.22	-0.937				-0.937			-0.937
7A	-2.37	-0.622			-0.622				-0.622
8A	-0.34	-0.322	-0.322		-0.322			-0.322	
9A	-1.54	-0.346	-0.346		-0.346			-0.346	
11A	-0.14	-0.041		-0.041		-0.041			-0.041
12A-M	-0.67	-0.371	-0.371			-0.371		-0.371	
12A-F	-0.98	-0.393		-0.393	-0.393			-0.393	
13A	0.00	-0.017			-0.017				-0.017
14A	0.41	0.236	0.236		0.236			0.236	
15A	0.32	0.174		0.174	0.174			0.174	
16A	-1.70	-0.699	-0.699		-0.699			-0.699	
17A-M	0.33	0.145	0.145				0.145	0.145	
17A-F	-0.18	-0.077		-0.077			-0.077	-0.077	
18A	-2.00	-0.631	-0.631			-0.631		-0.631	
19A	-1.94	-0.389				-0.389		-0.389	
21A	-0.60	-0.232	-0.232		-0.232			-0.232	
22A	-0.86	-0.250				-0.250			-0.250

C. MAS Scores

Study	Z	Mn-ES	ES-m	ES-f	ES-ya	ES-ma	ES-ea	ES-sur	ES-exp
4A	-1.54	-0.587	-0.587		-0.587				-0.587
5A	2.38	1.338	1.338			1.338			1.338
20A	0.00	0.000				0.000			0.000

Similarly, the method of calculating combined Z scores and conducting planned comparisons was the same as that described in chapter 6. A negative effect size and Z score each indicate a *decrease* in the dependent variable, whether measures of depression or anxiety. Our a priori predictions were that both depression and anxiety scores would show a decrease.

Results -- Depression Group

1. Main effects. As shown in Table 7.4, the combined effect of the studies in the depression group was a statistically significant decrease in depression scores, independent of instrument used to measure depression. The overall Z score was 9.296, with p<.00001.

2. Male-female differences. As shown in Table 7.3a, the gender of subjects was identified in only 10 of the 15 studies in the depression group. Nevertheless, of those that did report gender, it would appear that there was no significant difference between male and female groups in decreases in depression scores.

3. Age differences. Significant decreases in depression scores occurred in all age groups, that is, young, middle-aged, and elderly adults. The magnitude of the effect decreased monotonically across these age groups.

4. Survey versus experiment differences. Both the survey and the experiment reports in the depression group showed significant overall effects on depression, and the mean effect sizes for the two subgroups were not significantly different. Thus there were no differences as a function of the experimental rigor of the study.

5. Differences by type of exercise. As can be seen in the design summary in Table 7.2a, the type of exercise employed in all of the studies of the depression group was running/jogging. Therefore, no comparisons by type of exercise were possible in the depression group.

Table 7.4. Depression and anxiety groups -- Z scores, mean effect
        sizes (first row) and standard errors (second row)
        for each significant effect.

Measure Zst	Mn-ES	ES-m	ES-f	ES-ya	ES-ma	ES-ea	ES-sur	ES-exp
Depression								
N = 17 -9.296	-0.967	-1.093	-0.657	-1.156	-0.796	-0.715	-1.132	-0.899
p<.00001	0.182	0.356	0.379	0.253	0.456	0.313	0.357	0.218
Anxiety-state								
N = 13 -3.425	-0.279	-0.155	-0.308	-0.271	-0.595	0.000	-0.101	-0.432
p<.0003	0.095	0.075	0.343	0.117	0.182	--	0.077	0.144
Anxiety-trait								
N = 20 -3.569	-0.254	-0.283	-0.067	-0.247	-0.437	-0.049	-0.223	-0.313
p<.0002	0.070	0.103	0.092	0.108	0.127	0.077	0.083	0.133
MAS								
N = 3 0.485								
N.S.								

Results -- Anxiety Group

1. Main effects. As can be seen in Table 7.4, the combined effect on measures of STAI anxiety-state was statistically significant, with Z score = 3.425 and p<.0003. Similarly, the overall effect on STAI anxiety-trait was significant, with Z score = 3.569 and p<.0002. However comparisons with the MAS were not significant, hence no further comparisons with the MAS were made, and all considerations in the anxiety group will be limited to the STAI data.

2. Male-female differences. Both the anxiety-state and anxiety-trait decreases were observed in male groups. Female groups, however, did not show changes in either anxiety-state or anxiety-trait that were significantly greater than zero, and the anxiety-trait changes were also significantly less than those observed in male groups. In other words, the overall significant decreases in anxiety-state and anxiety-trait were produced almost exclusively by male groups. It can be seen, for example in Table 7.3b that there were only two cases of notable female negative effect sizes for anxiety-state and anxiety-trait combined.

3. Age differences. The significant decreases in both anxiety-state and anxiety-trait were observed in both young adult and middle-aged adults, but not in elderly adults. In this case the cause of this failure to find an effect is not necessarily due to the paucity of data, since there were five elderly groups that contributed to the overall effect size for anxiety-trait, as shown in Table 7.3b.

4. Survey versus experiment differences. The mean effect sizes for survey and experiment studies were significantly different for anxiety-state, but not anxiety-trait. In the case of anxiety-state, it was the survey studies that produced the lower effect size, which at least shows that the less rigorous studies did not produce the overall statistical significance for this measure.

5. Differences by type of exercise. There is no evidence that any one form of exercise produced any greater or lesser effect in the anxiety group.

Additional Comparisons

Several additional comparisons were also made at this point. Since the authors of the studies in the depression group used five different measures of depression, an opportunity was thus presented to test whether there were systematic differences between these instruments. Similarly, six of the groups summarized in Table 7.2a were in fact depressed subjects (indicated by asterisk), as opposed to normal volunteers, and of course there is great interest in testing whether or not the net effects on depression scores were different in such groups. (Unfortunately, none of the groups in the anxiety group were "anxious" subjects.) The results of these additional comparisons are summarized in Table 7.5.

As can be seen in Table 7.5, Part A, the five measures of depression appeared to differ in mean effect size. The Lubin DACL produced the largest mean effect size, although this result stems largely from two survey reports from the same laboratory. Furthermore, although the mean effect sizes for the Zung SDS and the Beck DI were not significantly different, there were differences in consistency of findings. That is, effect sizes in studies in which the Beck DI was used all fell within a narrow range, whereas similar studies in which the Zung SDS was used included one study in which no effect was found and one study in which an *increase* in depression was found. Thus, on detailed comparison of findings, a case can be made to suggest that the Beck DI has to date proved to be the most useful measure of depression in this group.

Table 7.5, Part B, shows the difference in mean effect size for the "normal" versus "depressed" groups. It can be seen that the mean effect size in the depressed groups (1.168) was about 40% larger than that seen in the normal groups (0.827), although still not a significant difference.

Table 7.5, Parts C to E, provides a summary of mean effect sizes by method of calculation for the depression group and the anxiety group, respectively. It can be seen that there were no systematic effects, although effect sizes calculated with norm data were significantly larger in the depression group, and smaller (but not significant) in the two anxiety groups. Even though this is an anomalous

Table 7.5. Additional data showing differences between (A) depression scales, (B) normal vs depressed subjects, and (C-E) the methods of calculating effect size.

	No. of studies	Mean effect size	Standard error
A. Depression scale			
1. Zung	7	-0.658	0.350
2. Beck	5	-1.215	0.173
3. Lubin	3	-1.540	0.362
4. CES-D	2	-0.733	0.733
5. SCL-90	1	-1.018	--
B. Normal vs. depressed subjects, depression group			
1. Normal	10	-0.827	0.254
2. Depressed	7	-1.168	0.254
C. Method of calculating effect size, depression group			
1. Full formula	6	-0.865	0.404
2. Glass formula	1	-0.939	--
3. Using t, F, etc.	7	-0.786	0.221
4. Using norm data	3	-1.605	0.298
D. Method of calculating effect size, anxiety-state group			
1. Full formula	2	-0.620	0.374
2. Glass formula	0	--	--
3. Using t, F, etc.	6	-0.298	0.141
4. Using norm data	5	-0.121	0.091
E. Method of calculating effect size, anxiety-trait group			
1. Full formula	3	-0.103	0.074
2. Glass formula	4	-0.174	0.128
3. Using t, F, etc.	8	-0.391	0.116
4. Using norm data	5	-0.191	0.175

Note: Effect sizes were calculated by either (1) full formula, (2) Glass formula, (3) derived from another statistic, such as t, F, etc., or (4) by using norm data in place of an absent control group.

finding, it is not viewed as influencing the results in any systematic manner.

General Findings -- Depression Studies

In general, the findings in the depression group may be summarized as follows:

1. The combined effect of all studies in this group indicated that there was a statistically significant decrease in depression scores, independent of instrument used to measure depression.

2. Decreases in depression scores were observed in both male and female groups. The difference between males and females was not statistically significant.

3. Significant decreases in depression scores occurred in all adult age groups, although the magnitude of the effect decreased monotonically from young adults, through middle age, to elderly adults.

4. There were no differences between survey and experiment reports, indicating no difference in observed effect as a function of rigor.

5. All of the studies in the depression group employed running/jogging as the form of exercise, hence no comparisons across types of exercise were possible.

6. Each of the five questionnaires used to measure depression appeared to be acceptably useful. However, there was some indication that the Beck DI was the most useful measure of depression in this group.

7. The decrease in depression was approximately 40% greater in depressed groups compared to normal subjects. Closer examination of the studies of depressed subjects indicated that the "confounds interpretation" of the results is less plausible than the interpretation that fitness training itself produced the effect.

8. Effect sizes calculated with norm data were significantly larger in the depression group. This was considered to be a secondary matter, since it involved only 3 of the 17 groups, and the overall

effects produced by other methods of calculation were still substantial.

General Findings -- Anxiety Studies

The primary findings in the anxiety group may be summarized as follows:

1. There was a statistically significant decrease on anxiety-state and anxiety-trait scores.
2. There was no significant effect on MAS scores.
3. The significant decreases in anxiety-state and anxiety-trait scores occurred almost exclusively in the male groups, with little effect noted in female groups.
4. Both young adults and middle-aged adults showed the significant decreases in state and trait anxiety, but not elderly adults, although all age groups were represented enough to determine if there was any effect at all.
5. There was no evidence to indicate that the significance of the results was unduly caused by the contribution of the survey studies.
6. Four different forms of exercise were employed by the investigators. There was no persuasive evidence that any one form of exercise was more effective. The majority used running/jogging/walking, and there was one each of cycling, dance, and mixed conditioning.
7. There were six groups of depressed subjects in the depression group, but there were too few comparable groups of anxious subjects in the anxiety group. Therefore, comparisons between so-called clinical and normal control groups were not possible. Obviously, further work on this question could be of great interest.
8. It was concluded that there was no systematic influence on the results due to the method of calculating effect sizes.

Depression and Anxiety Compared

On the basis of the foregoing analyses, it is possible to make some overall concluding statements about the effects of aerobic fitness training on depression and anxiety:

1. Aerobic fitness training produces a statistically significant decrease in depression, anxiety-state, and anxiety-trait, measures that are presumably both mood and trait.
2. The net effect size in the depression group was significantly greater than that in the anxiety group, indicating that the decrease in depression scores was greater than the decrease in anxiety-state and anxiety-trait scores.
3. There were no systematic gender differences in depression score changes, however, the decreases in anxiety-state and anxiety-trait were produced primarily by male groups.
4. Young and middle-aged adults demonstrated the decreases in both depression and anxiety, whereas elderly adults demonstrated the decrease in depression scores only.
5. There were no systematic differences between survey studies and experiment studies in effect on depression, anxiety-state, or anxiety-trait scores.
6. The decrease in depression scores was approximately 40% greater in depressed groups, thus supporting the frequent use of fitness programs as a treatment aid for depression. There was no indication that these results could be better explained as due to extraneous variables.
7. Some case can be made to suggest that the Beck DI has been the most useful measure of depression in fitness studies, although several others appear to be acceptable. Only one measure of anxiety-state and anxiety-trait was used in the studies reviewed.
8. No single method of calculating effect sizes contributed systematically to produce the observed results.

Interpretation of Findings for Depression and Anxiety

Probably the most interesting findings in these groups were (a) that there were significant effects on depression, anxiety-state, and anxiety-trait; (b) that the effects on depression were greater than the effects on anxiety-state and anxiety-trait; and (c) that the effects on depressed subjects were approximately 40% greater than those on normals.

Another interesting comparison is that between the two present groupings and the POMS mood group data described in chapter 6, especially using the depression and tension scores of the POMS. By comparing Table 6.5 and Table 7.4, it can be seen quickly that the overall effects on the POMS tension scores and the anxiety-state and anxiety-trait scores were very much the same, suggesting that the POMS tension scores and STAI anxiety-state and anxiety-trait data gave the same overall result.

Further inspection reveals, however, that this similarity of findings did not hold for depression scores. The POMS depression score was significantly lower than the overall effect size for the combined depression group, and also significantly lower than the "normals" in the depression group. Nevertheless, it would still appear that, in a broad sense, the results of the analysis of the mood group, and the results of the analysis of the depression and anxiety groups are quite similar, since, in both cases, we can conclude that an effect of aerobic fitness training has been demonstrated on an important aspect of mood.

It is also well established that aerobic fitness training is associated with a significant reduction in depression, a reduction that is approximately 40% greater in depressed subjects. Even though it is tempting to conclude that this relatively large effect size in depressed groups is a product of the problem confounds (expectancy effects, statistical regression, and spontaneous remission), closer inspection suggests that this may not be the wisest choice. There are several compelling reasons for this statement. First, all of the studies using depressed subjects (see Table 7.2a) were either true (3D, 4D, 7D, and 8D) or quasi-experiments (2D and 15D). Untreated or "waiting list" depressed controls were used in four studies (3D, 4D, 7D, and 15D), and in several cases the subjects were not told that they were participating in a study of depression. Consequently, in these studies the opportunity for expectancy effects, statistical regression, and spontaneous remission were apparently equal in both experimental and control groups, thus rendering the "confounds interpretation" less plausible than the interpretation that the effect was produced by the independent variable, namely, aerobic fitness training.

More critically, we were dismayed to find how often previous investigators omitted essential items in their reports. A number of the studies in the depression and anxiety groups failed to specify the gender of their subjects. Others left us to resort to guesswork to estimate the mean age of groups. Follow-up data were almost never collected. The great majority of studies was concerned with effects in young adult males. Studies with female subjects, plus middle-aged and elderly (male or female) subjects, were notably less frequent. Depressed subjects were used in six studies, however, there were no comparable reports with clinically anxious subjects. Such obvious gaps could provide a fruitful area for future efforts.

Lastly, we prefer to postpone discussion of the theoretical association between fitness training and effects on depression and anxiety until chapter 10.

Summary

This review of the studies on the effects of aerobic fitness training on depression and anxiety may be summarized as follows:

1. Depression and anxiety studies were selected to review separately because of the potential therapeutic value of effects on these aspects of mood, although a distinction can be made between state versus trait. The former implies a transient aspect of mood, whereas the latter suggests some more enduring characteristic.

2. Standardized tests used to measure depression and anxiety were described, including information on strengths and problems. Tests used to measure depression were the Beck DI, the CES-D Scale, the Lubin DACL, the SCL-90, and the Zung SDS. Tests

used to measure anxiety were the STAI and the MAS.

3. The depression group and the anxiety group were both described, including subject groups(s), mean age, experimental design, type of effect size, fitness exercise, and measure of fitness.

4. The results of the meta-analyses of both groups were presented, including main effects, sex differences, age differences, and differences by type of experimental design, type of effect size, and type of fitness exercise.

5. Differences between measures of depression and between depressed and nondepressed subjects were also presented.   No comparisons between anxious and nonanxious subjects could be made.

6. Significant effects were found for depression, anxiety-state, and anxiety-trait scores.   The observed effects on depression were greater than those on anxiety-state and anxiety-trait, and the effects on depressed subjects were nearly 40% greater than those on nondepressed subjects.   The data support the conclusion that this effect was produced primarily by aerobic fitness training, rather than known confounds.

7. These results were shown to be consistent with the results of the meta-analysis of the POMS studies presented in chapter 6, in the broad sense that both showed a significant effect on mood.

8. Several frequent or consistent errors of omission were noted in previous reports, such as missing or vague mention of gender and age of subjects, lack of follow-up data, and the dominant preference for young adult males as subjects, as opposed to other age groups, plus females.

EIGHT

SELF-CONCEPT STUDIES

This chapter is a review and analysis of the studies of the effects of aerobic fitness training on self-concept. Self-concept is generally defined as one's view or perception of oneself, or more simply how one sees oneself. This then includes terms such as self-awareness, self-image, self-knowledge, and also possibly self-ideal and self-esteem, although these latter terms more narrowly refer to the individual's perception of how he/she "ought" to be, a more evaluative judgment.

Such distinctions are not clearly or consistently made by writers in the field, and consequently there is some confusion in use of terms and possible risk of misinterpretation of published findings. We have therefore elected to use the term "self-concept" throughout this chapter, even though other authors have used terms such as self-esteem, real-self, body cathexis, and the like.

Similarly, one's total self-concept can be considered to be composed of parts, such as physical self-concept, social self-concept, moral self-concept, and so on; however, we have not judged such distinctions to be useful for purposes of the present review, and we have chosen the most global or total measure of self-concept whenever reported, regardless of which secondary measures might have been reported in addition.

This is not only logically consistent, but also reflects the most frequent practice of other investigators. For example, even though some scales include a number of subscores or components of self-concept, the so-called "total" score is most often the only one reported. In other cases where no such total score is reported, we have chosen the single score that is closest to "physical" self-concept or body cathexis because we are studying the effects of aerobic fitness training. In no case did we use two or more scores from a single sample in the self-concept group because of the nonindependence of such data.

Self-concept is regarded as a relatively stable characteristic of individuals, making it more trait-like or enduring.   The results of the present review are therefore
potentially of greater interest than the mood studies reviewed in chapter 6 if it can be shown that aerobic fitness
training does in fact have an effect on   more trait-like
characteristics, similar to the anxiety-trait data reported
in chapter 7.

Measures of Self-concept

Thirteen different instruments were used by investigators to measure self-concept effects.   Starting with the
most frequently reported, these instruments are: the Tennessee Self-Concept Scale (TSCS, 16 reports); the Coopersmith Self-Esteem Inventory (SEI, 5 reports); the Secord
and Jourard Body Cathexis Scale (4 reports); the Sonstroem
Physical Estimation and Attraction Scale (PEAS, 3 reports),
Piers-Harris Children's Self-Concept Scale (CSCS, 3 reports), and the Rosenberg Self-Esteem Scale (SES, 3 reports); the Bills Index of Adjustment and Values (2 reports),
Gough and Heilbrun Adjective Check List (ACL, 2 reports),
and the Osgood Semantic Differential (2 reports); and the
Benjamin Structural Analysis of Social Behavior, Emory
My Body Index. Jorgenson Social Vocabulary Index, and the
Pflaum Life Quality Inventory (1 report each).

Although these scales are superficially similar in. that
all scales attempt to measure self-concept, self-esteem,
physical self-concept, body cathexis, or similar concepts,
they vary widely in degree of standardization, reported
norm data, established reliability and validity, and critical
review in third party sources.   Therefore there will be similar differences in demonstrated utility in assessing fitness
training effects.   As an additional note of caution, scales
that have been used in only one or two studies should be
considered   as something less than fully established, even
in cases where significant effects were demonstrated.

Fitts Tennessee Self-Concept Scale
The standardized test of self-concept used most frequently in the self-concept group, the TSCS was developed
by Fitts (1965).   It consists of 100 statements that subjects

rate 1-5 for "completely false" to "completely true." Half of the statements are positive (e.g., I have a healthy body) and half are the opposite (e.g., I am a sick person). Responses are scored 1-5 for endorsing positive items, and 5-1 for not endorsing the negative items. These scores are then summed to yield a "total positive" score, which "reflects the overall level of self-esteem" (p. 2). Fitts apparently sees nothing inconsistent with the total score on a self-concept scale as reflecting self-*esteem*, and we and most others have interpreted the total positive score as something akin to global self-concept. Items are also clustered for scoring on a number of additional subscales, including "physical self-concept." However, as pointed out by Fitts, the correlations among these subscales are high (generally above .75; p. 16), and consequently we (along with most other investigators) have chosen to limit the analysis to the total positive score, which we label as total self-concept, primarily for convenience. Evaluative reviews of the TSCS have been written by Bentler (1972) and by Suinn (1972).

Coopersmith Self-Esteem Inventory

The Coopersmith SEI, in its adult form, consists of 25 items. There are five subscales, including a "general self" score, which we have chosen to use exclusively in the meta-analysis. Extensive findings on reliability and validity have been reported by Coopersmith (1967, 1981). The SEI has gained wide use as a research instrument in both child and adult groups, although less so than the TSCS.

Secord and Jourard Body Cathexis Scale

The Body Cathexis Scale developed by Secord and Jourard (1953) consists of 46 body parts and functions (e.g., hair, eyes, feet, sleep, exercise, etc.) that subjects are instructed to rate 1-5, reflecting "have strong feelings and wish could change" to "consider myself fortunate." We assume that the Secord-Jourard body cathexis score is similar to Fitts' physical self-concept score, but something less than a global measure of self-concept. However, Secord and Jourard report that body cathexis scores correlated .58 and .66 with a measure of self-cathexis in males and females, respectively.

Sonstroem Physical Estimation and Attraction Scale

The PEAS, developed by Sonstroem (1974, 1978), consists of 100 true-false statements that are scored for two primary scales: estimation (Est) and attraction (Attr), designed to measure physical self-concept and interest in physical activities, respectively. Sample items from each scale are: "I am stronger than a good many of my friends" (Est), and "I love to run" (Attr). In studies where the full PEAS was reported, we have selected only the estimation scale score for analysis.

Piers-Harris Children's Self-Concept Scale

The Piers-Harris CSCS (Piers & Harris, 1984) is one of the few self-concept questionnaires designed exclusively for children. It consists of 80 statements in yes-no format. There is a "total" score, which we have chosen to use in the meta-analysis, plus six subscales. A critical review has been published by Epstein (1985).

Rosenberg Self-Esteem Scale

The Rosenberg SES has been described by Rosenberg (1963). It consists of 10 statements (e.g., "On the whole, I am satisfied with myself"), and subjects are asked to rate each item from "strongly agree" to "strongly disagree."

Bills Index of Adjustment and Values

The Bills Index of Adjustment and Values was developed by Bills, Vance, and McLean (1951). The index is based on a Q-sort of a list of 124 trait words that subjects rate from 1-5, reflecting "seldom" to "most of the time" to measure self-concept. Several additional scores can be obtained, concerned with self-acceptance and ideal self. Bills et al. also report information on reliability and validity.

Gough and Heilbrun Adjective Check List

The Gough-Heilbrun ACL was originally introduced by Gough (1955, 1960), and further developed by Heilbrun (1958, 1959). It consists of 300 adjectives, and subjects are instructed to check all that apply. There are 24 scales from the total check list, including self-confidence, which we assume to be similar to self-esteem. Critical reviews of the Gough-Heilbrun ACL have been written by Rorer (1972), Vance (1972), Teeter (1985), and by Zarske (1985).

Osgood Semantic Differential

The Osgood Semantic Differential is a generic rating system introduced by Osgood, Suci, and Tannenbaum (1957) in which subjects rate a specified concept (such as "self" and "normal person") over 25 dimensions.   A variety of scores and difference scores can be obtained.

Other self-concept scales

The remaining four self-concept scales were reported in one study each in the self-concept group. For additional information, the reader is referred to the following: (1) Benjamin Structural Analysis of Social Behavior (see Benjamin, 1974); (2) Emory My Body Index (see Emory, 1980); (3) Jorgenson Social Vocabulary Index (see Jorgenson, Jansen, and Samuelson, 1968); and (4) Pflaum Life Quality Inventory (see Pflaum, 1973).

For more information about any of the scales listed above, the reader is also referred to the original research articles of the self-concept group for description on use of these scales.   Identification of what scale was used in which study may be made through Table 8.1 below.

Independent Variables

Thirty-seven studies were identified that met all selection criteria and constitute the self-concept group. The 37 studies, including identification number (alphabetical by first author), authors, year of publication, and self-concept scale used are given in Table 8.1.   Nine of the studies listed in Table 8.1 were included in the mood group (see Table 6.1), namely, Folkins (1976), Folkins et al. (1972), Kowal et al. (1978), McDonald et al. (1991), Morgan and Pollock (1977), Nagy and Frazier (1988), Perri and Templer (1984-85), Rudy and Estok (1983), and Wilfley and Kunce (1986).   Four of the studies in Table 8.1 were part of the depression group (see Table 7.1a), namely, Klein et al. (1985), Morgan and Pollock (1977), Parent and Whall (1984), and Perri and Templer (1984-85).   Lastly, four of the studies listed in Table 8.1 were also included in the   anxiety

Table 8.1. Self-concept group, showing identification
           number, authors, year of publication, and
           self-concept scale used.

ID	Authors	Year	Scale
1SC	Blackman, Hunter, Hilyer, and Harrison	1988	Coopersmith, Secord-Jourard and TSCS
2SC	Bolton and Milligan	1976	TSCS
3SC	Brinkmann and Hoskins	1979	Jorgenson
4SC	Brown, Morrow, and Livingston	1982	TSCS
5SC	Collingwood and Willett	1971	Bills
6SC	Collingwood	1972	Bills
7SC	Dodson and Mullens	1969	Osgood
8SC	Eickhoff, Thorland, and Ansorge	1983	TSCS
9SC	Folkins	1976	Secord-Jourard
10SC	Folkins et al.	1972	Gough-Heilbrun
11SC	Gary and Guthrie	1972	Secord-Jourard
12SC	Hanson and Nedde	1974	TSCS
13SC	Hilyer and Mitchell	1979	TSCS
14SC	Joesting and Clance	1979	Secord-Jourard
15SC	Klein et al.	1985	Benjamin
16SC	Kowal et al.	1978	PEAS
17SC	Leonardson and Gargiulo	1978	Osgood
18SC	MacMahon and Gross	1987	Piers-Harris
19SC	Maloney et al.	1986	Coopersmith
20SC	Marsh and Peart	1988	Rosenberg
21SC	McDonald et al.	1991	TSCS & PEAS

(table continues)

(Table 8.1, continued)

ID	Authors	Year	Scale
22SC	McGowan, Jarman, and Pedersen	1974	TSCS
23SC	Morgan and Pollock	1977	PEAS
24SC	Morris and Husman	1978	Pflaum
25SC	Nagy and Frazier	1988	Coopersmith
26SC	Netz et al.	1988	TSCS
27SC	Parent and Whall	1984	Rosenberg
28SC	Pauly et al.	1982	TSCS
29SC	Percy, Dziuban, and Martin	1981	Coopersmith
30SC	Perri and Templer	1984-85	TSCS
31SC	Plummer and Koh	1987	TSCS
32SC	Riddick and Freitag	1984	Emory
33SC	Rudy and Estok	1983	Rosenberg
34SC	Sherrill, Holguin, and Caywood	1989	Piers-Harris
35SC	Short, DiCarlo, Steffee, and Pavlou	1984	TSCS
36SC	Wilfley and Kunce	1986	TSCS
37SC	Young	1985	TSCS

group (see Table 7.1b), namely, Kowal et al. (1978), Maloney et al. (1986), Morgan and Pollock (1977), and Netz et
al. (1988).

Specific design characteristics of the studies in the
self-concept group are given in Table 8.2. Following the
same format used in chapters 6 and 7, Table 8.2 gives the
following information for each study: identification number, number of groups, number of subjects per group,
number of male and female subjects, mean age, experimental design and type of effect size, fitness exercise,
and measure(s) of fitness.   Male and female data are reported separately in the reports by Folkins et al. (1972),
Maloney et al. (1986), Netz et al. (1988), and Sherrill et
al. (1989), hence these groups are treated as two studies
in the meta-analysis.   Gaps in the gender and age columns
indicate information that was not specifically reported by
the authors. In some cases, it was still possible to estimate
the subjects' age (e.g., if the subjects were described as
college freshmen).   The rating systems for experimental
design and type of effect size are described in detail in
chapter 6.

Results by Study

Z scores and effect sizes for each study in the self-
concept group are summarized in Table 8.3.   The column
headings in Table 8.3 are the same as those used in chapters 6 and 7.   The dependent variable for each study in
Table 8.3 was the effect size calculated from a single
measure of self-concept, regardless of instrument.   This
information therefore constitutes the raw data for the
meta-analysis of the self-concept group, and it is given at
this point primarily to facilitate the repeatability of our
analysis, plus any additional analyses that the reader may
wish to pursue.

Results by Group

Results of the meta-analysis of the self-concept group
are summarized in Table 8.4, based entirely on the raw

Table 8.2. Self-concept group, independent variables.

Study	No. Grps	Ne	Nc	Nm	Nf	Age	Design/ ES-type	Fitness Exercise	Measure of Fitness
1SC	2	8	8	--	16	15.3	4/1	dance	VO2max, BP, %BF
2SC	1	12	--	12	--	20	2/2	walk/jog	step test, wt, 60-yd run
3SC	1	7	--	2	5	43.7	2/3	bike	HR, bike ergometer
4SC	2	50	50	--	100	22	12/3	jog	1.5-m run, body comp.
5SC	1	5	--	5	--	15?	2/3	jog	HR, Kraus Weber series
6SC	2	25	25	50	--	20?	4/3	jog	step test, Kraus Weber
7SC	1	18	--	14	4	35?	1/3	jog	BP, body composition
8SC	2	20	19	--	39	27?	4/1	dance	HR, bike ergometer
9SC	2	18	18	36	--	50?	4/2	walk/jog	BP, HR, lipids
10SC	2	42	42	42	42	19?	10/2	jog	HR, 1.75-m run
11SC	2	10	10	20	--	40	4/3	jog	HR
12SC	1	8	--	--	8	28	2/2	walk/jog	treadmill, bike ergometer
13SC	2	80	40	77	43	19.8	4/3	run	12-min run
14SC	2	56	14	70	--	20?	3/3	runners	running history
15SC	2	14	14	--	--	30?	4/1	run/walk	program completion
16SC	1	85	--	85	--	20?	2/2	basic training	%BF, VO2max

(table continues)

Table 8.2, continued.

Study	No. Grps	Ne Nc	Nm Nf	Age	Design/ ES-type	Fitness Exercise	Measure of Fitness
17SC	1	15 --	-- --	18?	2/2	jog	12-min run
18SC	2	27 27	54 --	9.7	4/1	run/dance	bike ergometer
19SC	1	43 --	15 28	31.0	1/2	run	step test, 2 mi run
20SC	2	-- --	-- 137	13	4/3	dance	step test
21SC	1	92 --	-- --	27.7	1/3	military training	VO2max
22SC	2	37 --	37 --	12?	4/3	run	12-min run
23SC	1	27 --	27 --	24.8	1/4	elite runners	VO2max
24SC	2	20 31	36 15	20	3/1	run	1.5-m run
25SC	2	31 54	-- 85	21.4	3/2	dance	exercise history
26SC	1	24 --	11 13	58	2/2	walk/jog	treadmill, HR
27SC	1	30 --	-- --	60+	3/3	mixed	self-report
28SC	1	73 --	-- --	36	2/3	run/bike	%BF, HR, VO2max
29SC	2	15 15	-- --	10?	4/3	run	running history
30SC	2	23 19	14 28	65.4	10/3	walk/jog	compulsory class
31SC	2	116 177	-- 293	22	10/2	dance	class completion
32SC	2	6 8	-- 14	65+	3/3	dance+	class completion

(table continues)

(Table 8.2, continued)

Study	No. Grps	Ne Nc	Nm Nf	Age	Design/ ES-type	Fitness Exercise	Measure of Fitness
33SC	1	319 --	-- 319	35?	1/3	10k/ marathon	running history
34SC	2	52 52	52 52	10	1/2	exercise history	1-mi run
35SC	2	22 23	45 --	40?	4/3	walk/jog	treadmill
36SC	2	49 34	-- --	43.0	10/2	walk/run	lap run
37SC	2	128	-- 128	14?	1/3	exercise history	600-yd run

Note: HR = heart rate, %BF = percent body fat, BP = blood pressure.

Table 8.3. Self-concept studies, Z scores and effect sizes.

Study	Z	Mn-ES	ES-m	ES-f	ES-ya	ES-ma	ES-ea	ES-sur	ES-exp
1SC	0.31	0.500		0.500	0.500				0.500
2SC	-1.10	-0.485	-0.485		-0.485			-0.485	
3SC	2.01	2.099				2.099		2.099	
4SC	1.72	0.354		0.354	0.354				0.354
5SC	2.52	2.321	2.321		2.321			2.321	
6SC	1.96	0.585	0.585		0.585				0.585
7SC	2.25	1.259				1.259		1.259	
8SC	1.11	0.373		0.373	0.373				0.373
9SC	-0.83	-0.290	-0.290			-0.290			-0.290
10SC-M	0.72	0.231	0.231		0.231				0.231
10SC-F	2.82	1.012		1.012	1.012				1.012
11SC	0.96	0.469	0.469			0.469			0.469
12SC	2.22	1.350		1.350	1.350			1.350	
13SC	2.22	0.606			0.606				0.606
14SC	2.51	0.633	0.633		0.633			0.633	

(table continues)

(Table 8.3, continued)

Study	Z	Mn-ES	ES-m	ES-f	ES-ya	ES-ma	ES-ea	ES-sur	ES-exp
15SC	2.47	1.048			1.048				1.048
16SC	2.19	0.340	0.340		0.340			0.340	
17SC	0.57	0.218			0.218			0.218	
18SC	0.79	0.222	0.222		0.222				0.222
19SC-M	0.49	0.267	0.267			0.267		0.267	
19SC-F	0.83	0.331		0.331	0.331			0.331	
20SC	1.03	0.177		0.177	0.177				0.177
21SC	1.71	0.382			0.382			0.382	
22SC	1.69	0.591	0.591		0.591				0.591
23SC	2.81	0.659	0.659		0.659			0.659	
24SC	2.41	0.725			0.725			0.725	
25SC	2.41	0.551		0.551	0.551			0.551	
26SC-M	0.33	0.144	0.144				0.144	0.144	
26SC-F	0.23	0.097		0.097			0.097	0.097	
27SC	3.70	1.214					1.214	1.214	
28SC	2.68	0.473				0.473		0.473	
29SC	2.94	1.302			1.302				1.302
30SC	2.40	0.811					0.811		0.811
31SC	1.96	0.230		0.230	0.230				0.230
32SC	1.28	0.783		0.783			0.783	0.783	
33SC	0.00	0.000		0.000	0.000			0.000	
34SC-M	2.33	0.687	0.687		0.687			0.687	
34SC-F	0.57	0.163		0.163	0.163			0.163	
35SC	0.98	0.305	0.305			0.305			0.305
36SC	-0.29	-0.065				-0.065			-0.065
37SC	2.00	0.298		0.298	0.298			0.298	

data given in Table 8.3.   All column headings in Table 8.4
are the same as those used in chapters 6 and 7.   In addition, the method of calculating combined Z scores and
conducting planned comparisons was the same as that described and used in chapters 6 and 7.   A positive ES and
Z score both indicate an *increase* in the dependent variable,
the chosen measure of self-concept.   Our a priori prediction
was that all measures of self-concept would show an increase.

Results -- Self-concept Group

1. Main effects. As shown in Table 8.4, the total combined
effect of aerobic fitness training in the self-concept group
was a statistically significant increase in self-concept
scores, independent of the scale or instrument used to
measure self-concept.   The overall Z score was 9.669, with
p<.00001.

2. Male-female differences. As can be seen in Table 8.3,
25 of the 37 studies in the self-concept group identified
the gender of their subjects in sufficient detail to permit
calculation of effect sizes.   Of those that did report gender, it would appear that both male and female subjects
showed a resulting increase in self-concept, and there is
no significant difference in the effect sizes of males and
females shown in Table 8.4

3. Age differences. Significant increases in self-concept
scores occurred in all age groups, that is, young, middle-
aged, and elderly adults.   The magnitude of the effect increased monotonically across the age groups, as can be seen
in Table 8.4, with the elderly group showing the largest
effect size.

4. Survey versus experiment differences. Both the survey
and the experiment reports in the self-concept group
showed significant overall effects on self-concept, and the
mean effect sizes for the two subgroups were similar (0.631
and 0.470, respectively).   Thus the overall findings in the
survey studies and the experiment studies were nearly the
same, indicating no differences in findings as a function
of the experimental rigor of the study.

Table 8.4. Self-concept group, Z score, mean effect sizes
(first row) and standard error (second row).

Measure Zst	Mn-ES	ES-m ES-f	ES-ya ES-ma ES-ea	ES-sur ES-exp
Self-concept				
N = 41 9.669	0.560	0.445 0.444	0.550 0.565 0.610	0.631 0.470
p<.00001	0.087	0.160 0.100	0.098 0.272 0.214	0.136 0.093

Table 8.5. Additional data showing differences between
(A) self-concept scales and (B) the methods of
calculating effect size.

	No. of studies	Mean effect size	Standard error
A. Self-Concept scale			
1. TSCS	16	0.342	0.100
2. Coopersmith	5	0.530	0.202
3. Secord-Jourard	4	0.229	0.205
4. PEAS	3	0.541	0.101
5. Piers-Harris	3	0.357	0.166
6. Rosenberg	3	0.464	0.379
7. Bills	2	1.453	0.868
8. Gough-Heilbrun	2	0.622	0.391
9. Osgood	2	0.739	0.521
10. Others*	4	1.164	0.320
B. Method of calculating effect size			
1. Full formula	5	0.574	0.144
2. Glass formula	16	0.299	0.112
3. Using t, F, etc.	19	0.772	0.142
4. Using norm data	1	0.659	--

Note: Effect size was calculated by either (1) full formula,
(2) Glass formula, (3) derived from another statistic,
such as t, F, etc., or (4) by using norm group data
in place of an absent control group.
*Other measures reported (each in one study only) were the
Benjamin, Emory, Jorgenson, and Pflaum scales.

5. *Differences by type of exercise.* As shown in Table 8.2, most of the studies in the self-concept group employed running/jogging exercise programs. There were six studies that used aerobic dance, and one study that used bike exercise exclusively. Two studies used a complex combination. The mean effect size for the six studies that used dance (0.436) was similar to the overall mean for the self-concept group, and therefore not significantly different from the running/jogging studies. The effect in the one study to use bike exercise is too small for comparison with the remainder.

Additional Comparisons

Several additional comparisons were made at this point. Because the investigators in the self-concept group used 13 different measures of self-concept (including self-esteem, body cathexis, and the like), we were presented with an opportunity to compare the average effect sizes across instruments and form a judgment about the relative homogeneity (or vice versa) of the group. In addition, as was also true in chapters 6 and 7, we were concerned about possible effects produced by the fact that effect sizes were calculated by four different methods, and we wanted to determine whether or not this difference in statistical procedure had any bearing on the results of the meta-analysis.

As shown in Part A of Table 8.5, the 13 self-concept instruments are listed by frequency of use within the self-concept group, beginning with the most frequently used instrument, the TSCS, and ending with a cluster of tests that were each used only once, labeled "Other." The mean effect sizes of the three scales (Bills, Gough-Heilbrun, and Osgood) reported in only two studies each clearly should be disregarded at this time as potentially unreliable. Of the remaining six instruments, three (the TSCS, Coopersmith, and PEAS) show the largest mean effect sizes relative to the standard errors, suggesting that one of these scales would likely be more useful in future studies. Some investigators may of course wish to choose a given instrument on some other basis, such as greater comparability with other studies, as in using the TSCS.

Part B of Table 8.5 provides a summary of mean effect sizes by method of calculation for the self-concept group. It can be seen that there was only one case of an effect size calculated from norm data. The mean effect size in the group based on the original Glass formula was significantly lower than one other group, however, this would not appear to be a source of systematic error.

General Findings

In general, the findings in the self-concept group may be summarized as follows:

1. The combined effect of all studies in this group indicated that there was a statistically significant increase in self-concept scores, independent of the instrument used to measure self-concept.
2. Increases in self-concept scores were observed in both male and female groups. The difference in overall effect between males and females was not statistically significant.
3. Similarly, increases in self-concept scores were observed in all age groups, that is, young, middle-aged, and elderly adults.
4. The differences between the survey and experiment reports were not significant, indicating that the experimental rigor of the study had no effect on the outcome of the meta-analysis.
5. There were no indications that the form of exercise had any effect on the outcome of the meta-analysis, although this was largely a result of the fact that most of the studies (28 out of 37) studied running/jogging/walking as the form of exercise.
6. There were no indications that the instrument used to measure self-concept had any effect on the results, although there was great variability in the frequency of use of tests. One (the TSCS) was reported in 16 studies, and the remaining 12 instruments reported were used in 1-5 studies. In spite of the foregoing, there was some basis for recommending either the TSCS, Coopersmith, or PEAS in future studies.

7. There were no systematic effects on the results solely as a function of method of calculating effect size.

Interpretation of Findings

Doubtless the most important finding from the meta-analysis of the effect of aerobic fitness training on measures of self-concept is that there is indeed a highly significant and positive effect on self-concept, independent of the scale used to measure self-concept. By "self-concept," we include a small list of related concepts, such as self-esteem, physical self-concept, body cathexis, and real-self. All of these measures show similar positive effects of aerobic fitness training.

One can also compare the results of the meta-analysis of self-concept studies with the results of the depression and anxiety studies by comparing Table 7.4 with Table 8.4 It can be seen that the effect size for the self-concept group is significantly greater than both anxiety-state and anxiety-trait, but significantly less than depression (disregarding sign). Therefore the overall effect in both the self-concept and depression groups was greater than in the anxiety group, although the findings for self-concept were significantly less than those for depression.

This result is especially significant when one further considers that self-concept is a relatively trait-like or enduring characteristic of the individual, certainly more enduring than the mood measures reported in chapter 6 and the depression and anxiety-state measures reported in chapter 7. Self-concept is probably more similar to the anxiety-trait measures reported in chapter 7, however, the fact that self-concept by its very nature is intended to be a more global construct makes the self-concept findings of greater long-term interest than the anxiety-trait findings. That is, we consider the self-concept findings to be potentially the most enduring result to date when compared with the mood and anxiety-trait data of previous chapters. However, few of the studies reported to date included follow-up data. The findings are limited to those changes that occur after 10 to 15 weeks of fitness training, and there is no information on the lasting impact of fitness

training after 6 or 12 months, an obvious gap in the existing literature that needs to be filled.   One exception is
the project reported by Hanson and Nedde (1974), who
studied the effects of fitness training over a period of 8
months and found a substantial effect on TSCS total score.
More studies of this duration are seriously needed.

It is also of interest to note that the effect on self-
concept is apparently the same in (a) males and females,
(b) all age groups, (c) survey reports and experiment studies, and (d) all studies regardless of the method used to
compute the effect size.

Of great potential interest was the finding that there
was a significant positive effect in all age groups, that is,
young, middle-aged, and elderly adults.   This should serve
to stimulate further studies of the effects of fitness
training in elderly groups, especially when it is also noted
that studies of elderly groups *in general* in fitness studies
make up a very small percent of the total number of studies.   Most studies have been concerned with effects in
young adult groups, generally close to age 20, and we expect that this bias will continue for some significant period
of time.

As a concluding note, we were again dismayed to find
that the quality of reporting within the self-concept group
was highly variable, quite similar to the problem noted in
previous chapters.   Inspection of Table 8.2 shows the
number of studies that did not report the gender and/or
age of subjects.   In Table 8.3, it can be seen that in 12
out of 37 studies, the investigators did not report gender
data completely enough to assign an effect size to either
the male or female column.   Numerous other gaps occurred.
In one case, an instrument was described in the Methods
section of a report and then never mentioned again.   In
several instances, the only clue we had that there was a
statistical analysis at all was a single cryptic "p<.05" given
parenthetically at the end of a concluding statement.   In
other cases, the data were reported inconsistently, so that,
for example, one study was included in the mood group of
chapter 6 because of the information reported, but failed
to qualify for the self-concept group of chapter 8, even
though there was brief mention that a self-concept questionnaire was administered.   Our goal in calling attention
to these problems is of course to improve the quality of

reporting in the future, rather than engage in criticism for its own sake. This is an important matter to which we return in chapter 10.

Summary

Our meta-analysis of the studies of the effects of aerobic fitness training on self-concept may be summarized as follows:

1. Self-concept is defined as a relatively enduring or trait-like characteristic of the individual, in contrast to more transient states, such as mood or depression and anxiety. Because self-concept is defined in relatively global terms, it is also viewed as more enduring than the anxiety-trait studies reviewed in chapter 7. *earlier*

2. Self-concept is generally defined as the manner in which one views oneself, and therefore includes a variety of similar terms, such as self-knowledge, self-awareness, and so on. In addition, although the formal definition of self-esteem is more narrow, referring to how one *ought* to be, the distinction is not made consistently in the literature, and we have included this concept within the rubric of self-concept. Similarly, various component parts of global self-concept, most notably physical self-concept, have been shown to correlate highly with total scores, and therefore we have not found it practical to maintain the distinction.

3. Thirteen instruments were used to measure self-concept (and related concepts) in the 37 studies in the self-concept group. The TSCS was used in 16 studies, and each of the remainder was used in 1 to 5 studies.

4. The self-concept group was described, including each of the following where available: subject group(s), number of males and females per group, mean age, experimental design, type of effect size, fitness exercise, and measure of fitness.

5. The results of the meta-analysis were presented, including main effect, gender differences, age dif-

ferences, and differences by type of experimental design, effect size, fitness exercise, and measure of self-concept employed.

6. Significant overall and positive effects on self-concept were found, independent of the measure of self-concept employed. The effect on self-concept was found to be significantly greater than both anxiety-state and anxiety-trait, but significantly less than depression, as reported in chapter 7. easily

7. There were no meaningful differences due to gender, age, rigor of the study, fitness exercise used, or method of calculating effect size. Significant overall effects were found in all of these subgroups. There were indications that the TSCS, Coopersmith, and PEAS measures of self-concept may be more recommended in future studies.

8. The significance of these results was discussed and compared to the findings reported in previous chapters.

9. Problems created by incomplete and/or ambiguous literature reports were noted. Several areas of improvement and needed future work were discussed.

NINE

PERSONALITY STUDIES

In this chapter, we present a critical review of the studies of the effects of aerobic fitness training on measures of personality. In this instance, the measures of personality to be reported are those derived from various objective personality questionnaires or inventories. Most of these inventories range from under 100 to over 500 items, often in true-false format, which in turn produce scores on a number of scales in the form of a profile. Investigators can (and often do) select individual scales to administer as a shortened form of the total inventory without difficulty.

In general, the questionnaires are based on a fundamentally trait-defined view of personality, and the scale scores are therefore intended to measure some combination of personality traits. The traits, in turn, are usually defined as relatively *enduring* habit patterns. For example, subjects are typically instructed to respond in terms of "what is most usually true" or how they feel "in general," rather than "today" or "this week."

The intent of this chapter therefore is to assess the effects of aerobic fitness training on the most enduring measures employed in the existing literature, in contrast to more transient constructs, such as mood, anxiety, or depression, which were reviewed in previous chapters. We make no assumption about the validity of the underlying personality theory (if any) on which a given instrument may be based, but rather we concern ourselves solely with the question of whether or not a scale is sensitive to the effects of aerobic fitness training. Consideration of the underlying theory in general has been postponed until chapter 10.

As an aside, we note that not all measures derived from personality inventories actually constitute enduring personality traits, an important consideration in the analysis to follow. For example, the depression scale on the Minnesota Multiphasic Personality Inventory (MMPI) is an obvious example of a scale that can show relatively large change in a short time in response to acute upset, therapeutic intervention, and so on, regardless of the instructions to respond in terms of what is true "in general." This is an important point to which we return later.

Measures of Personality

A total of nine different personality inventories has been reported in studies that we found to be otherwise acceptable for inclusion in our review. However, six of these inventories were used in one to three reports only. This was no problem in previous chapters, because tests that produce correlated or highly overlapping scores can be combined in a meta-analysis, as was done in chapter 8 with 13 different measures of self-concept. Personality inventories, however, are not so monolithic as tests of self-concept, and consequently we found it necessary to drop the studies where investigators used the underrepresented instruments. Instead we confined ourselves only to those instruments where there was an adequate number of studies on which to base our meta-analysis.

The result of this selection process was a final group in which three personality inventories were adequately represented for purposes of a meta-analysis. These three inventories, listed alphabetically, are the Cattell Sixteen Personality Factor Questionnaire (16PF; 16 groups in 14 reports), the Eysenck Personality Inventory (EPI; 12 groups in 11 reports), and the Minnesota Multiphasic Personality Inventory (MMPI; 8 groups in 8 reports). There were two reports in which both the 16PF and EPI were used, plus two reports in which two separate exercise groups were studied, and these are therefore treated separately in the meta-analysis. Similarly, since the three personality inventories (16PF, EPI, and MMPI) produce nonoverlapping scale scores, it was necessary to conduct a separate meta-analysis for each scale for each inventory, over as many scales as the inventory produces. The resulting increased risk of Type I error in testing for statistical significance of our results is a question to which we return.

The 16PF, EPI, and MMPI have each existed for a number of years, and consequently each has generated an extensive research literature that far exceeds our available space and purposes here. The following summary description is intended only for introductory or refresher purposes. The interested reader who wishes a more complete background is strongly encouraged to consult any of the many available sources on this topic.

Sixteen Personality Factor Questionnaire

The personality inventory most represented in our personality group is the 16PF. The inventory was originally developed by Raymond Cattell in 1949, although there have since been several revisions (see Cattell, Eber, & Tatsuoka, 1970). Based solely on an extensive factor analysis, the 16PF, as the name implies, is intended to measure 16 different source traits, as opposed to surface traits. The test consists of 187 items presented in multiple-choice format, most (but not all) with choices such as "yes," "in between," "no," or "agree," "uncertain," "no." Some items have a right or wrong answer, but most do not. There are 16 bipolar scales, with the following common labels for scores at the high end of the scale: A-warmth, B-intelligence, C-emotional stability, E-dominance, F-impulsivity, G-conformity, H-boldness, I-sensitivity, L-suspicious, M-imagination, N-shrewdness, O-insecurity, Q1-radicalism, Q2-self-sufficiency, Q3-self-discipline, and Q4-tension.

The 16PF, more than most other personality inventories, has been the target of a number of highly critical reviews. Relatively positive reviews have been published by Bolton (1978) and Wittenborn (1953), whereas more negative conclusions have been expressed by Bloxom (1978), Harsh (1953), Lubin (1953), Walsh (1978), and Zuckerman (1985). In addition, Digman and Takemoto-Chock (1981), and Digman and Inouye (1986) have indicated that some of Cattell's data (derived in a precomputer age) suffer from computational errors. Lastly, the data of Digman and colleagues suggest that there is little empirical justification for 16 separate factors, as opposed to their framework of 5 primary factors. Nevertheless, as pointed out by Butcher (1985):

> The 16PF, developed as a research instrument for assessing source traits, seems to be gaining in application for normal range assessment situations in

recent years. The 16PF is most valuable as a personality measure in settings such as personnel selection, guidance counseling, or personality research, where assessment of "normal range" personality traits is important. (p. 1392)

In general, our experience, in finding the 16PF to be the most frequently used personality inventory in fitness research, would seem to correspond highly with Butcher's observation.

Eysenck Personality Inventory
   The EPI was developed by Eysenck and Eysenck (1963). There have been several earlier versions (e.g., the Maudsley Personality Inventory), as well as a more recent revision (the Eysenck Personality Questionnaire; EPQ), generally occasioned by the addition of new scales. However, we confine our descriptive comments to the one form of the test represented in the meta-analysis, namely, the EPI. The EPI provides scores on two primary scales: neuroticism (N; 23-24 items) and extraversion (E; 21-24 items). Response format is "yes, true" or "no, not true." There is also a lie scale (L; 21 items), however, most investigators have not included this scale in their reports, generally because high scores are quite atypical in the groups studied. Therefore our meta-analysis of the EPI studies consists solely of the N and E scales. Reviews of these scales, whether based on the EPI or the EPQ, have been written by Tellegen (1978), Block (1978), Kline (1978), and Stricker (1978). Most reviewers have noted some encouraging properties of the N and E scales, while still voicing some frustrations over unanswered questions about the ultimate utility of the scales. Interestingly, Noller, Law, and Comrey (1987) have reported that the N and E scales show high factor loadings on two of the five robust factors reported by Digman and colleagues.

Minnesota Multiphasic Personality Inventory
   The MMPI (Hathaway and McKinley, 1943) is probably the oldest and most used of the so-called objective personality inventories. It consists of over 500 items in true/false format, although the use of abbreviated forms (and fewer scale scores) is practical and commonplace.

The ten clinical scales are: hypochondriasis (Hs; 33 items), depression (D; 60 items), hysteria (Hy; 60 items), psychopathic deviate (Pd; 50 items), masculinity-femininity (Mf; 60 items), paranoia (Pa; 40 items), psychasthenia (Pt; 48 items), schizophrenia (Sc; 78 items), hypomania (Ma; 46 items), and social introversion (Si; 70 items).   There are also three validity scales (termed the L, F, and K scales), although, like the lie scale on the EPI, high scores are very atypical, and therefore most investigators did not report the data from these validity scales, and our meta-analysis is confined to the clinical scales.   For a more detailed discussion of the questions of scale validity, item overlap, and so on, the interested reader is referred to any of the more lengthy sources, such as Dahlstrom, Welsh, and Dahlstrom (1972-1975) or Anastasi (1982).

It should be noted that the MMPI is intended for clinical assessment with relatively disordered clinical groups rather than the normal population, and this is reflected in some of the individual items (e.g., "My soul sometimes leaves my body"), as well as the recommended profile interpretations.   This characteristic of the MMPI was probably in Butcher's mind when he made the observation (quoted above) that the 16PF, unlike the MMPI, has gained in recent years in use for "normal range assessment."   One result of this difference in questionnaire bias is that nearly all of the MMPI studies in our personality group were studies in which the groups chosen for evaluation were those with demonstrated medical or behavioral diagnoses, placing them outside of the normal range, and creating questions of comparability in the interpretation of our findings.   This is a matter to which we return below.

Independent Variables

Thirty-one studies were identified that met all of the selection criteria and constitute the personality group.   The 31 studies, including identification number (alphabetical by first author), authors' names, year of publication, and personality inventory used are given in Table 9.1. Five of the studies listed in Table 9.1 were included in the mood group (see Table 6.1), namely, Carney et al. (1983), Kowal et al. (1978), Morgan et al. (1987, 1988), and Suominen-Troyer

Table 9.1. Personality group, showing identification
number, authors, year of publication, and
personality inventory used.

ID	Authors	Year	Inventory
1P	Buccola and Stone	1975	16PF
2P	Carney et al.	1983	MMPI
3P	Dodson and Mullens	1969	MMPI
4P	Dulberg and Bennett	1980	16PF
5P	El-Naggar	1986	EPI
6P	Frankel and Murphy	1974	MMPI
7P	Hammer and Wilmore	1973	16PF
8P	Hartung and Farge	1979	16PF
9P	Ismail and Young	1973	16PF
10P	Ismail and Young	1977	16PF and EPI
11P	Jasnoski and Holmes	1981	16PF
12P	Jette	1975	16PF
13P	Johnson et al.	1985	EPI
14P	Jones and Weinhouse	1979	16PF
15P	Kavanagh, Shephard, Tuck, and Qureshi	1977	MMPI
16P	Kowal et al.	1978	EPI
17P	Lobstein, Mosbacher, and Ismail	1983	MMPI
18P	Mikel	1983	EPI
19P	Morgan and Costill	1972	EPI
20P	Morgan et al.	1988	EPI
21P	Morgan et al.	1987	EPI
22P	Morgan and Pollock	1977	EPI

(table continues)

(Table 9.1, continued)

ID	Authors	Year	Inventory
23P	Naughton, Bruhn, and Lategola	1968	MMPI
24P	Renfrow and Bolton	1979	16PF
25P	Sharp and Reilley	1975	MMPI
26P	Stern and Cleary	1981	MMPI
27P	Suominen-Troyer et al.	1986	EPI
28P	Tillman	1965	16PF
29P	Valliant, Bennie, and Valiant	1981	16PF
30P	Vanfraechem and Vanfraechem-Raway	1978	16PF
31P	Young and Ismail	1976	16PF and EPI

et al. (1986). Three of the studies in Table 9.1 were part of the depression group (see Table 7.1a), namely, Jasnoski and Holmes (1981), Morgan and Costill (1972), and Morgan and Pollock (1972). Four of the studies in Table 9.1 were part of the anxiety group (see Table 7.1b), namely, Hammer and Wilmore (1973), Johnson et al. (1985), and Morgan et al. (1987, 1988). And one of the studies in Table 9.1 was included in the self-concept group (see Table 8.1), namely, Dodson and Mullens (1969).

Specific design characteristics of the studies in the personality group are given in Table 9.2 for the 16PF, EPI, and MMPI groups, respectively. The following information for each group is included: identification number, number of groups, number of subjects per group, number of male and female subjects, mean age, experimental design and type of effect size, fitness exercise, and measure(s) of fitness. Buccola and Stone (1975) studied two different exercise groups, and Young and Ismail (1976) studied two different age groups, hence in both of these cases the data are treated as two studies in the meta-analysis. In addition, Ismail and Young (1977) and Young and Ismail (1976) used both the 16PF and the EPI, and therefore each inventory is included in the respective subgroups. Question marks in the age column in Table 9.2 indicate information that was not specifically given by the investigators, but, in some cases, estimated from statements made in the text of the article.

There are several additional problems with the EPI and MMPI groups. Firstly, and most importantly, the EPI and MMPI groups consist primarily, but not entirely, of survey studies. There are two experiment studies in the EPI group (27P and 31P) and in the MMPI group (2P and 23P).

To compound the problem, in one case (2P) the authors reported only three of the MMPI scales, and in the other (23P) the authors simply reported that the MMPI data were "not significant," in which case we used effect sizes of 0.000 for all scales. In addition, in all but two of the studies in the MMPI group, the groups consisted of clinical samples (rather than "normal range" groups), for example, hemodialysis patients, psychiatric patients, alcoholics, and three studies of postcoronary patients. Obviously, these considerations must limit our capacity for general conclu-

Table 9.2. Independent variables.

Study	No. of Groups	Ne	Nc	Nm	Nf	Age	Design/ ES-type	Fitness Exercise	Measure of Fitness

a. 16PF Studies

Study	No. of Groups	Ne	Nc	Nm	Nf	Age	Design/ ES-type	Fitness Exercise	Measure of Fitness
1P-A	1	20	--	20	--	70?	2/3	cycling	BP, bike ergometer, VO2max
1P-B	1	16	--	16	--	70?	2/3	jog	see 1P-A
4P	2	30	30	60	--	15?	10/3	jog	program completion
7P	2	9	9	18	--	30?	10/2	jog	VO2max,
8P	1	48	--	48	--	47.4	1/4	run/jog	VO2max, HR, %BF
9P	2	14	14	28	--	40's	10/1	run/jog	VO2max, BP, %BF
10P	1	58	--	58	--	43.2	2/2	run/jog	VO2max, BP, %BF
11P	1	103		--	103	20.3	2/3	run+	12-min run
12P	2	23	21	44	--	49	3/2	run/jog	Cureton program
14P	1	12	--	7	5	30.3	2/3	run	HR, BP, bike ergometer
24P	2	23	23	46	--	43	3/2	run/jog	exercise history
28P	2	63	50	113	--	17?	3/2	run/jog	Cureton program
29P	1	30	--	30	--	34.4	1/4	marathon	history of marathon
30P	2	10	10	--	20	13	10/1	bike	bike ergometer
31-A	2	7	7	14	--	32	10/2	run/jog	VO2max

(table continues)

(Table 9.2, continued)

Study	No. of Groups	Ne	Nc	Nm	Nf	Age	Design/ ES-type	Fitness Exercise	Measure of Fitness
31-B	2	7	7	14	--	51	10/2	run/jog	VO2max

b. EPI Studies

Study	No. of Groups	Ne	Nc	Nm	Nf	Age	Design/ ES-type	Fitness Exercise	Measure of Fitness
5P	1	30	--	30	--	45?	2/2	jog	VO2max
10P	See Table 9.2a								
13P	1	6	--	6	--	21	2/4	cycling	%BF, lipid VO2max
16P	1	85	--	85	--	20?	2/2	basic training	%BF, VO2max
18P	1	310	--	216	94	35.1	1/4	run	running history
19P	1	9	--	9	--	32	1/4	marathon	history of marathon
20P	1	14	--	14	--	26.4	1/4	running history	running history
21P	1	15	--	--	15	27.2	1/4	running history	running history
22P	1	27	--	27	--	24.8	1/4	elite runners	running history
27P	2	10	20	--	30	42.6	10/2	run/jog	HR, BP, BF
31-A&B	See Table 9.2a								

c. MMPI Studies

Study	No. of Groups	Ne	Nc	Nm	Nf	Age	Design/ ES-type	Fitness Exercise	Measure of Fitness
2P	2	4	4	6	2	40?	4/2	bike/jog	VO2max
3P	1	18	--	14	4	35?	1/3	jog	BP, body comp.
6P	1	214	--	214	--	45	2/2	walk/bike or row	HR, step test
15P	1	44	--	44	--	50?	2/2	jog	bike ergometer

(table continues)

(Table 9.2, continued)

Study	No. of Groups	Ne	Nc	Nm	Nf	Age	Design/ ES-type	Fitness Exercise	Measure of Fitness
17P	2	11	11	22	--	49	3/2	run	HR, BP, %BF, est VO2max
23P	2	14	14	28	--	48	10/2	jog	HR
25P	1	65	--	65	--	20?	1/3	run	VO2max, 12-min run
26P	1	618	--	618	--	45?	2/3	bike+	completed program

Note: Ne and Nc = number of subjects in the experimental and control groups; Nm and Nf = number of male and female subjects; Age = mean for the total group; BP = blood pressure, %BF = percent body fat, HR = heart rate.

sions based on the EPI and the MMPI groups, although one partial solution is suggested below.

Results by Study

Z scores and effect sizes for each study in the personality group are given in Tables 9.3 to 9.5. Table 9.3 summarizes the results for each scale of the 16PF; Table 9.4 for the EPI; and Table 9.5 for the MMPI. The column headings in these tables are the same as those used in previous chapters. The information therefore constitutes the raw data for the meta-analyses in the personality group, and it is given here to insure the repeatability of our analysis, plus any additional analyses that may be suggested.

Results by Group

Results of the meta-analysis for the personality group are summarized in Table 9.6 (a, 16PF studies; b, EPI studies; and c, MMPI studies). The column headings in these tables are the same as those used in previous chapters. In addition, the methods of calculating combined Z scores and conducting planned comparisons are the same as those first described in chapter 6. A negative ES and Z score both indicate a *decrease* in the mean scale score. Our a priori predictions were that mean scores on most scales would decrease as a result of aerobic fitness training, especially where such decreases indicate improved adjustment or reduction in behavior disorder symptomatology. This was clearly the case with the scales on the EPI and MMPI; however, there are several scales on the 16PF where score increases may be interpreted as indicative of improved functioning, most notably scales B (intelligence), C (emotional stability), Q2 (self-sufficiency), and Q3 (self-discipline). In these latter cases, we predicted an increase in mean scale scores, but a decrease in the mean scores on the remaining 16PF scales.

Table 9.3. 16PF studies -- Z scores and effect sizes as calculated for each study.

Study	Z	ES	ES-m	ES-f	ES-ya	ES-ma	ES-ea	ES-sur	ES-exp
a. A Scale (Warmth)									
1P-A	-1.26	-0.602	-0.602				-0.602	-0.602	
1P-B	0.94	0.505	0.505			0.505		0.505	
4P	2.23	0.608	0.608		0.608				0.608
7P	0.63	0.325	0.325			0.325			0.325
8P	-1.51	-0.461	-0.461			-0.461		-0.461	
9P	-0.87	-0.347	-0.347			-0.347			-0.347
11P	0.00	0.000		0.000	0.000			0.000	
12P	-1.01	-0.317	-0.317			-0.317		-0.317	
14P	0.85	0.536				0.536		0.536	
24P	-2.15	-0.684	-0.684			-0.684		-0.684	
28P	0.05	0.008	0.008		0.008			0.008	
29P	-1.99	-0.790	-0.790			-0.790		-0.790	
30P	0.96	0.465		0.465	0.465				0.465
31P-A	0.00	0.000	0.000			0.000			0.000
31P-B	0.00	0.000	0.000			0.000			0.000
b. B Scale (Intelligence)									
1P-A	-0.27	-0.124	-0.124				-0.124	-0.124	
1P-B	-0.45	-0.236	-0.236				-0.236	-0.236	
4P	2.33	0.891	0.891		0.891				0.891
7P	-0.25	-0.127	-0.127			-0.127			-0.127
8P	2.63	0.838	0.838			0.838		0.838	
9P	-0.60	-0.241	-0.241			-0.241			-0.241
11P	0.00	0.000		0.000	0.000			0.000	
12P	0.21	0.066	0.066			0.066		0.066	
14P	2.51	1.828				1.828		1.828	
24P	0.81	0.246	0.246			0.246		0.246	
28P	1.09	0.208	0.208		0.208			0.208	
29P	2.55	1.036	1.036			1.036		1.036	
30P	0.00	0.000		0.000	0.000				0.000
31P-A	1.01	0.610	0.610			0.610			0.610
31P-B	1.12	0.682	0.682			0.682			0.682

(table continues)

(Table 9.3, continued)

c. C Scale (Emotional Stability)

Study	Z	ES	ES-m	ES-f	ES-ya	ES-ma	ES-ea	ES-sur	ES-exp
1P-A	0.19	0.090	0.090				0.090	0.090	
1P-B	0.10	0.062	0.062				0.062	0.062	
4P	0.00	0.000	0.000		0.000				0.000
7P	-1.39	-0.742	-0.742			-0.742			-0.742
8P	0.47	0.139	0.139			0.139		0.139	
9P	-1.21	-0.491	-0.491			-0.491			-0.491
10P	0.56	0.150	0.150			0.150		0.150	
11P	0.00	0.000		0.000	0.000			0.000	
12P	-0.32	-0.098	-0.098			-0.098		-0.098	
14P	0.52	0.321				0.321		0.321	
24P	-0.17	-0.052	-0.052			-0.052		-0.052	
28P	1.63	0.313	0.313		0.313			0.313	
29P	0.00	0.000	0.000			0.000		0.000	
30P	1.18	0.581		0.581	0.581				0.581
31P-A	0.82	0.491	0.491			0.491			0.491
31P-B	1.08	0.658	0.658			0.658			0.658

d. E Scale (Dominance)

Study	Z	ES	ES-m	ES-f	ES-ya	ES-ma	ES-ea	ES-sur	ES-exp
1P-A	-0.86	-0.404	-0.404				-0.404	-0.404	
1P-B	1.56	0.865	0.865				0.865	0.865	
4P	2.91	0.864	0.864		0.864				0.864
7P	-1.99	-1.087	-1.087			-1.087			-1.087
8P	-0.17	-0.050	-0.050			-0.050		-0.050	
9P	0.13	0.052	0.052			0.052			0.052
10P	-0.49	-0.130	-0.130			-0.130		-0.130	
11P	0.00	0.000		0.000	0.000			0.000	
12P	-0.19	-0.060	-0.060			-0.060		-0.060	
14P	1.89	1.287				1.287		1.287	
24P	0.96	0.295	0.295			0.295		0.295	
28P	0.18	0.035	0.035		0.035			0.035	
29P	0.00	0.000	0.000			0.000		0.000	
30P	0.00	0.000		0.000	0.000				0.000
31P-A	0.45	0.268	0.268			0.268			0.268
31P-B	-1.11	-0.675	-0.675			-0.675			-0.675

(table continues)

(Table 9.3, continued)

e. F Scale (Impulsivity)

Study	Z	ES	ES-m	ES-f	ES-ya	ES-ma	ES-ea	ES-sur	ES-exp
1P-A	-0.27	-0.127	-0.127				-0.127	-0.127	
1P-B	-3.30	-2.099	-2.099				2.099	-2.099	
4P	0.00	0.000	0.000		0.000				0.000
7P	-0.14	-0.070	-0.070			-0.070			-0.070
8P	-2.15	-0.670	-0.670			-0.670		-0.670	
9P	-1.07	-0.430	-0.430			-0.430			-0.430
11P	0.00	0.000		0.000	0.000			0.000	
12P	-2.05	-0.663	-0.663			-0.663		-0.663	
14P	2.49	1.810				1.810		1.810	
24P	1.24	0.382	0.382			0.382		0.382	
28P	2.32	0.447	0.447		0.447			0.447	
29P	-0.39	-0.148	-0.148			-0.148		-0.148	
30P	0.87	0.423		0.423	0.423				0.423
31P-A	0.00	0.000	0.000			0.000			0.000
31P-B	0.00	0.000	0.000			0.000			0.000

f. G Scale (Conformity)

Study	Z	ES	ES-m	ES-f	ES-ya	ES-ma	ES-ea	ES-sur	ES-exp
1P-A	0.64	0.229	0.229				0.229	0.229	
1P-B	-0.58	-0.308	-0.308				-0.308	-0.308	
4P	0.00	0.000	0.000		0.000				0.000
7P	-1.75	-0.949	-0.949			-0.949			-0.949
8P	0.83	0.248	0.248			0.248		0.248	
9P	-1.39	-0.568	-0.568			-0.568			-0.568
10P	-0.23	-0.060	-0.060			-0.060		-0.060	
11P	0.00	0.000		0.000	0.000			0.000	
12P	0.81	0.253	0.253			0.253		0.253	
14P	0.69	0.431				0.431		0.431	
24P	-2.55	-0.824	-0.824			-0.824		-0.824	
28P	1.27	0.242	0.242		0.242			0.242	
29P	0.00	0.000	0.000			0.000		0.000	
30P	0.00	0.000		0.000	0.000				0.000
31P-A	-1.41	-0.882	-0.882			-0.882			-0.882
31P-B	1.41	0.885	0.885			0.885			0.885

(table continues)

(Table 9.3, continued)

g. H Scale (Boldness)

Study	Z	ES	ES-m	ES-f	ES-ya	ES-ma	ES-ea	ES-sur	ES-exp
1P-A	-0.20	-0.023	-0.023				-0.023	-0.023	
1P-B	1.18	0.639	0.639				0.639	0.639	
4P	2.20	0.600	0.600		0.600				0.600
7P	-1.44	-0.810	-0.810			-0.810			-0.810
8P	-1.04	-0.312	-0.312			-0.312		-0.312	
9P	-2.03	-0.864	-0.864			-0.864			-0.864
11P	0.00	0.000		0.000	0.000			0.000	
12P	-1.54	-0.491	-0.491			-0.491		-0.491	
14P	-0.66	-0.413				-0.413		-0.413	
24P	-0.89	-0.273	-0.273			-0.273		-0.273	
28P	1.14	0.220	0.220		0.220			0.220	
29P	0.00	0.000	0.000			0.000		0.000	
30P	0.00	0.000		0.000	0.000				0.000
31P-A	1.17	0.717	0.717			0.717			0.717
31P-B	0.86	0.404	0.404			0.404			0.404

h. I Scale (Sensitivity)

Study	Z	ES	ES-m	ES-f	ES-ya	ES-ma	ES-ea	ES-sur	ES-exp
1P-A	-1.03	-0.533	-0.533				-0.533	-0.533	
1P-B	1.82	1.026	1.026				1.026	1.026	
4P	1.82	0.403	0.403		0.403				0.403
7P	1.18	0.618	0.618			0.618			0.618
8P	-0.58	-0.174	-0.174			-0.174		-0.174	
9P	-0.05	-0.031	-0.031			-0.031			-0.031
11P	0.00	0.000		0.000	0.000			0.000	
12P	-2.08	-0.674	-0.674			-0.674		-0.674	
14P	-0.94	-0.594				-0.594		-0.594	
24P	-1.24	-0.382	-0.382			-0.382		-0.382	
28P	0.34	0.064	0.064		0.064			0.064	
29P	1.50	0.592	0.592			0.592		0.592	
30P	0.00	0.000		0.000	0.000				0.000
31P-A	0.00	0.000	0.000			0.000			0.000
31P-B	0.00	0.000	0.000			0.000			0.000

(table continues)

(Table 9.3, continued)

i. L Scale (Suspicious)

Study	Z	ES	ES-m	ES-f	ES-ya	ES-ma	ES-ea	ES-sur	ES-exp
1P-A	0.24	0.111	0.111				0.111	0.111	
1P-B	-0.14	-0.073	-0.073				-0.073	-0.073	
7P	0.10	0.057	0.057			0.057			0.057
8P	-0.83	-0.248	-0.248			-0.248		-0.248	
9P	-0.71	-0.282	-0.282			-0.282			-0.282
11P	0.00	0.000		0.000	0.000			0.000	
12P	-0.61	-0.191	-0.191			-0.191		-0.191	
14P	-0.53	-0.332				-0.332		-0.332	
24P	1.66	0.513	0.513			0.513		0.513	
28P	-0.52	-0.099	-0.099		-0.099			-0.099	
29P	0.00	0.000	0.000			0.000		0.000	
30P	0.00	0.000		0.000	0.000				0.000
31P-A	-1.72	-1.100	-1.100			-1.100			-1.100
31P-B	-1.45	-0.915	-0.915			-0.915			-0.915

j. M Scale (Imagination)

Study	Z	ES	ES-m	ES-f	ES-ya	ES-ma	ES-ea	ES-sur	ES-exp
1P-A	0.43	0.202	0.202				0.202	0.202	
1P-B	-0.68	-0.361	-0.361				-0.361	-0.361	
7P	-0.13	-0.064	-0.064			-0.064			-0.064
8P	2.08	0.645	0.645			0.645		0.645	
9P	-1.42	-0.583	-0.583			-0.583			-0.583
10P	-0.43	-0.115	-0.115			-0.115		-0.115	
11P	0.00	0.000		0.000	0.000			0.000	
12P	0.53	0.164	0.164			0.164		0.164	
14P	1.09	0.699				0.699		0.699	
24P	0.38	0.116	0.116			0.116		0.116	
28P	-1.29	-0.247	-0.247		-0.247			-0.247	
29P	1.74	0.691	0.691			0.691		0.691	
30P	0.00	0.000		0.000	0.000				0.000
31P-A	1.23	0.755	0.755			0.755			0.755
31P-B	1.83	1.181	1.181			1.181			1.181

(table continues)

(Table 9.3, continued)

Study	Z	ES	ES-m	ES-f	ES-ya	ES-ma	ES-ea	ES-sur	ES-exp
			k. N Scale (Shrewdness)						
1P-A	-0.68	-0.319	-0.319				-0.319	-0.319	
1P-B	0.93	0.498	0.498				0.498	0.498	
7P	-0.08	-0.053	-0.053			-0.053			-0.053
8P	1.31	0.397	0.397			0.397		0.397	
9P	0.00	0.000	0.000			0.000			0.000
10P	-0.31	-0.083	-0.083			-0.083		-0.083	
11P	0.00	0.000		0.000	0.000			0.000	
12P	1.04	0.327	0.327			0.327		0.327	
14P	-1.20	-0.774				-0.774		-0.774	
24P	-2.30	-0.724	-0.724			-0.724		-0.724	
28P	-0.64	-0.122	-0.122		-0.122			-0.122	
29P	-0.39	-0.148	-0.148			-0.148		-0.148	
30P	0.00	0.000		0.000	0.000				0.000
31P-A	0.00	0.000	0.000			0.000			0.000
31P-B	0.00	0.000	0.000			0.000			0.000
			l. O Scale (Insecurity)						
1P-A	0.33	0.154	0.154				0.154	0.154	
1P-B	0.70	0.371	0.371				0.371	0.371	
4P	0.00	0.000	0.000		0.000				0.000
7P	1.09	0.571	0.571			0.571			0.571
8P	-0.50	-0.149	-0.149			-0.149		-0.149	
9P	-1.35	-0.439	-0.439			-0.439			-0.439
10P	-0.30	-0.081	-0.081			-0.081		-0.081	
11P	-4.00	-1.120		-1.120	-1.120			-1.120	
12P	-0.13	-0.041	-0.041			-0.041		-0.041	
14P	-0.41	-0.250				-0.250		-0.250	
24P	0.40	0.123	0.123			0.123		0.123	
28P	-1.32	-0.254	-0.254		-0.254			-0.254	
29P	-0.52	-0.197	-0.197			-0.197		-0.197	
30P	0.00	0.000		0.000	0.000				0.000
31P-A	-1.15	-0.705	-0.705			-0.705			-0.705
31P-B	-1.50	-0.945	-0.945			-0.945			-0.945

(table continues)

(Table 9.3, continued)

m. Q1 Scale (Radicalism)

Study	Z	ES	ES-m	ES-f	ES-ya	ES-ma	ES-ea	ES-sur	ES-exp
1P-A	0.43	0.201	0.201				0.201	0.201	
1P-B	1.43	0.791	0.791				0.791	0.791	
7P	-0.39	-0.200	-0.200			-0.200			-0.200
8P	-0.65	-0.193	-0.193			-0.193		-0.193	
9P	0.29	0.116	0.116			0.116			0.116
11P	-3.80	-0.794		-0.794	-0.794			-0.794	
12P	0.79	0.246	0.246			0.246		0.246	
14P	-0.49	-0.303				-0.303		-0.303	
24P	3.03	1.032	1.032			1.032		1.032	
28P	0.36	0.068	0.068		0.068			0.068	
29P	0.00	0.000	0.000			0.000		0.000	
30P	0.00	0.000		0.000	0.000				0.000
31P-A	0.00	0.000	0.000			0.000			0.000
31P-B	0.00	0.000	0.000			0.000			0.000

n. Q2 Scale (Self-Sufficiency)

Study	Z	ES	ES-m	ES-f	ES-ya	ES-ma	ES-ea	ES-sur	ES-exp
1P-A	1.90	0.937	0.937				0.937	0.937	
1P-B	2.23	1.298	1.298				1.298	1.298	
4P	0.00	0.000	0.000		0.000				0.000
7P	0.00	0.000	0.000			0.000			0.000
8P	2.72	0.858	0.858			0.858		0.858	
9P	-1.45	-0.599	-0.599			-0.599			-0.599
11P	0.00	0.000		0.000	0.000			0.000	
12P	0.72	0.225	0.225			0.225		0.225	
14P	-0.74	-0.465				-0.465		-0.465	
24P	2.74	0.922	0.922			0.922		0.922	
28P	-4.00	-1.049	-1.049			-1.049		-1.049	
29P	2.33	0.938	0.938			0.938		0.938	
30P	0.00	0.000		0.000	0.000				0.000
31P-A	0.23	0.134	0.134			0.134			0.134
31P-B	2.03	1.336	1.336			1.336			1.336

(table continues)

(Table 9.3, continued)

Study	Z	ES	ES-m	ES-f	ES-ya	ES-ma	ES-ea	ES-sur	ES-exp
o. Q3 Scale (Self-Discipline)									
1P-A	0.78	0.366	0.366				0.366	0.366	
1P-B	-1.65	-0.912	-0.912				-0.912	-0.912	
4P	0.00	0.000	0.000		0.000				0.000
7P	-0.50	-0.256	-0.256			-0.256			-0.256
8P	0.52	0.154	0.154			0.154		0.154	
9P	-0.88	-0.354	-0.354			-0.354			-0.354
11P	0.00	0.000		0.000	0.000			0.000	
12P	-0.08	-0.220	-0.220				-0.220	-0.220	
14P	-0.66	-0.413				-0.413		-0.413	
24P	-1.16	-0.358	-0.358			-0.358		-0.358	
28P	-0.29	-0.056	-0.056		-0.056			-0.056	
29P	-0.39	-0.148	-0.148			-0.148		-0.148	
30P	0.00	0.000		0.000	0.000				0.000
31P-A	-0.10	-0.067	-0.067			-0.067			-0.067
31P-B	1.14	0.755	0.755			0.755			0.755
p. Q4 Scale (Tension)									
1P-A	-1.30	-0.621	-0.621				-0.621	-0.621	
1P-B	-1.94	-1.040	-1.040				-1.040	-1.040	
4P	0.00	0.000	0.000		0.000				0.000
7P	-0.29	-0.150	-0.150			-0.150			-0.150
8P	0.80	0.238	0.238			0.238		0.238	
9P	-0.15	-0.061	-0.061			-0.061			-0.061
10P	0.10	0.032	0.032			0.032		0.032	
11P	-2.42	-0.492		-0.492	-0.492			-0.492	
12P	-1.82	-0.561	-0.561			-0.561		-0.561	
14P	-1.88	-1.281				-1.281		-1.281	
24P	0.29	0.089	0.089			0.089		0.089	
28P	-1.99	-0.383	-0.383		-0.383			-0.383	
29P	0.00	0.000	0.000			0.000		0.000	
30P	0.00	0.000		0.000	0.000				0.000
31P-A	-0.80	-0.477	-0.477			-0.477			-0.477
31P-B	-2.11	-1.405	-1.405			-1.405			-1.405

Table 9.4. EPI studies --Z scores and effect sizes as
calculated for each study.

Study	Z	ES	ES-m	ES-f	ES-ya	ES-ma	ES-ea	ES-sur	ES-exp
					a. Extraversion Scale				
5P	-0.35	-0.131	-0.131				-0.131	-0.131	
10P	-0.43	-0.116	-0.116				-0.116	-0.116	
13P	-0.08	-0.050	-0.050		-0.050			-0.050	
16P	0.88	0.134	0.134		0.134			0.134	
18P	-3.75	-0.458					-0.458	-0.458	
19P	-1.09	-0.913	-0.913				-0.913	-0.913	
20P	0.36	0.203	0.203		0.203			0.203	
21P	0.92	0.512		0.512	0.512			0.512	
22P	0.22	0.088	0.088		0.088			0.088	
27P	0.00	0.000		0.000		0.000			0.000
31P-A	0.31	0.186	0.186				0.186	0.186	
31P-B	-1.14	-0.696	-0.696				-0.696	-0.696	
					b. Neuroticism Scale				
5P	-0.19	-0.073	-0.073				-0.073	-0.073	
10P	-0.15	-0.039	-0.039				-0.039	-0.039	
13P	-0.23	-0.221	-0.221		-0.221			-0.221	
16P	-1.28	-0.195	-0.195		-0.195			-0.195	
18P	-1.08	-0.128					-0.128	-0.128	
19P	0.10	0.093	0.093				0.093	0.093	
20P	-0.25	-0.143	-0.143		-0.143			-0.143	
21P	0.52	0.287		0.287	0.287				
22P	0.18	0.071	0.071		0.071			0.071	
27P	0.00	0.000		0.000		0.000			0.000
31P-A	-0.32	-0.187	-0.187				-0.187	-0.187	
31P-B	-1.37	-0.856	-0.856				-0.856	-0.856	

Table 9.5. MMPI studies -- Z scores and effect sizes as calculated for each study.

a. Hypochondriasis Scale (Hs)

Study	Z	ES	ES-m	ES-f	ES-ya	ES-ma	ES-ea	ES-sur	ES-exp
2P	-0.60	-0.522				-0.522			-0.522
3P	-2.11	-1.136				-1.136		-1.136	
6P	-3.35	-0.470	-0.470			-0.470		-0.470	
15P	-1.53	-0.484	-0.484			-0.484		-0.484	
17P	-0.98	-0.453				-0.453		-0.453	
23P	0.00	0.000				0.000			0.000
25P	-2.14	-0.558	-0.558		-0.558			-0.558	

b. Depression Scale (D)

Study	Z	ES	ES-m	ES-f	ES-ya	ES-ma	ES-ea	ES-sur	ES-exp
2P	0.20	0.174				0.174			0.174
3P	0.00	0.000				0.000		0.000	
6P	-4.00	-0.687	-0.687			-0.687		-0.687	
15P	-2.61	-0.853	-0.853			-0.853		-0.853	
17P	-2.13	-1.046				-1.046		-1.046	
23P	0.00	0.000				0.000			0.000
25P	-1.74	-0.449	-0.449		-0.449			-0.449	
26P	-3.74	-0.313	-0.313			-0.313		-0.313	

c. Hysteria Scale (Hy)

Study	Z	ES	ES-m	ES-f	ES-ya	ES-ma	ES-ea	ES-sur	ES-exp
2P	0.20	0.174				0.174			0.174
3P	0.00	0.000				0.000		0.000	
6P	-4.00	-0.666	-0.666			-0.666		-0.666	
15P	-1.77	-0.560	-0.560			-0.560		-0.560	
17P	1.44	0.681				0.681		0.681	
23P	0.00	0.000				0.000			0.000
25P	-2.14	-0.558	-0.558		-0.558			-0.558	

d. Psychopathic Deviate Scale (Pd)

Study	Z	ES	ES-m	ES-f	ES-ya	ES-ma	ES-ea	ES-sur	ES-exp
3P	0.00	0.000				0.000		0.000	
6P	-3.09	-0.454	-0.454			-0.454		-0.454	
15P	-0.62	-0.190	-0.190			-0.190		-0.190	
17P	0.27	0.123				0.123		0.123	
23P	0.00	0.000				0.000			0.000
25P	0.05	0.020	0.020		0.020			0.020	

(table continues)

(Table 9.5, continued)

Study	Z	ES	ES-m ES-f	ES-ya ES-ma ES-ea	ES-sur ES-exp

e. Masculine-Feminine Scale (Mf)

Study	Z	ES	ES-m	ES-f	ES-ya	ES-ma	ES-ea	ES-sur	ES-exp
3P	0.00	0.000				0.000		0.000	
6P	0.00	0.000	0.000			0.000		0.000	
15P	-0.37	-0.115	-0.115			-0.115		-0.115	
17P	0.05	0.016				0.016		0.016	
23P	0.00	0.000				0.000			0.000
25P	-0.95	-0.240	-0.240		-0.240			-0.240	

f. Paranoia Scale (Pa)

Study	Z	ES	ES-m	ES-f	ES-ya	ES-ma	ES-ea	ES-sur	ES-exp
3P	0.00	0.000				0.000		0.000	
6P	-2.65	-0.363	-0.363			-0.363		-0.363	
15P	-0.20	-0.060	-0.060			-0.060		-0.060	
17P	0.00	0.000				0.000		0.000	
23P	0.00	0.000				0.000			0.000
25P	-0.71	-0.180	-0.180		-0.180			-0.180	

g. Psychasthenia Scale (Pt)

Study	Z	ES	ES-m	ES-f	ES-ya	ES-ma	ES-ea	ES-sur	ES-exp
3P	-2.09	-1.124				-1.124		-1.124	
6P	-3.80	-0.599	-0.599			-0.599		-0.599	
15P	-1.05	-0.325	-0.325			-0.325		-0.325	
17P	-0.87	-0.398				-0.398		-0.398	
23P	0.00	0.000				0.000			0.000
25P	-3.78	-1.148	-1.148		-1.148			-1.148	

h. Schizophrenia Scale (Sc)

Study	Z	ES	ES-m	ES-f	ES-ya	ES-ma	ES-ea	ES-sur	ES-exp
3P	0.00	0.000				0.000		0.000	
6P	-3.60	-0.499	-0.499			-0.499		-0.499	
15P	-0.66	-0.203	-0.203			-0.203		-0.203	
17P	0.73	0.333				0.333		0.333	
23P	0.00	0.000				0.000			0.000
25P	-3.10	-0.842	-0.842		-0.842			-0.842	

(table continues)

(Table 9.5, continued)

Study	Z	ES	ES-m	ES-f	ES-ya	ES-ma	ES-ea	ES-sur	ES-exp
i. Hypomania Scale (Ma)									
3P	0.00	0.000				0.000		0.000	
6P	1.19	0.167	0.167			0.167		0.167	
15P	-0.55	-0.170	-0.170			-0.170		-0.170	
17P	0.54	0.246				0.246		0.246	
23P	0.00	0.000				0.000			0.000
25P	1.41	0.364	0.364		0.364			0.364	
j. Social Introversion Scale (Si)									
3P	0.00	0.000				0.000		0.000	
6P	-1.97	-0.273	-0.273			-0.273		-0.273	
15P	-0.31	-0.094	-0.094			-0.094		-0.094	
17P	-2.52	-1.248				-1.248		-1.248	
23P	0.00	0.000				0.000			0.000
25P	-3.35	-0.894	-0.894		-0.894			-0.894	

16PF

1. Main effects. As shown in Table 9.6a, 4 of the 16 scales showed significant effects: scale B (intelligence; $Z = 3.168$), O (insecurity; $Z = -2.165$), Q2 (self-sufficiency; $Z = 2.249$), and Q4 (tension; $Z = -3.378$). As indicated by the Z scores, mean scores on intelligence and self-sufficiency increased, whereas mean scores on insecurity and tension decreased, all at better than $p<.02$ and in the predicted direction. In other words, the meta-analysis of the 16PF studies shows that aerobic fitness training produces significant increases in 16PF scale scores on intelligence and self-sufficiency, and decreases in scale scores on insecurity and tension.

2. Male-female differences. Male groups generally dominated in the 16PF studies, making most gender comparisons difficult and tentative. In general, the significant effects on intelligence and self-sufficiency were observed only in male groups. There was some suggestion of effects on insecurity and tension in females, however, this comparison will need to be repeated at a later date in order to establish 16PF effects in females.

3. Age differences. Young and middle-aged adults showed reliable changes in scores on intelligence, insecurity, and tension, but inconsistent effects on self-sufficiency. Elderly adults, in contrast, showed marked and highly significant effects in both self-sufficiency and tension, but an opposite effect on intelligence and insecurity, that is, changes in the opposite direction of those seen in the two younger groups. These data indicate that age differences may play a significant role in any effort to assess personality effects of aerobic fitness training.

4. Survey versus experiment differences. By applying our usual criterion that mean effect sizes differ reliably from each other only when the difference is greater than two standard errors, it is clear that the mean effect sizes in the survey studies were not significantly different from the experiment studies in scores on the four 16PF scales, namely, intelligence, insecurity, self-sufficiency, and tension.

Table 9.6.   Z scores and mean effect sizes (first row) and standard
errors (second row) for scales showing significant
effects.

Measure	Zst	Mn-ES	ES-m	ES-f	ES-ya	ES-ma	ES-ea	ES-sur	ES-exp

a. 16PF Studies

Measure	Zst	Mn-ES	ES-m	ES-f	ES-ya	ES-ma	ES-ea	ES-sur	ES-exp
A-scale N = 15	-0.808 N.S.								
B-scale N = 15	3.168 p<.0008	0.378 0.152	0.321 0.136	0.000 --	0.275 0.211	0.549 0.217	-0.180 0.056	0.429 0.225	0.303 0.196
C-scale N = 16	0.865 N.S.								
E-scale N = 16	0.818 N.S.								
F-scale N = 15	-0.633 N.S.								
G-scale N = 16	-0.565 N.S.								
H-scale N = 15	-0.323 N.S.								
I-scale N = 15	0.191 N.S.								
L-scale N = 14	-1.205 N.S.								
M-scale N = 15	1.348 N.S.								

(table continues)

(Table 9.6, continued)

Measure	Zst	Mn-ES	ES-m	ES-f	ES-ya	ES-ma	ES-ea	ES-sur	ES-exp
N-scale N = 15	-0.599 N.S.								
O-scale N = 16	-2.165 p<.015	-0.185 0.112	-0.122 0.114	-0.560 0.560	-0.344 0.266	-0.211 0.134	0.263 0.109	-0.144 0.126	-0.253 0.225
Q1-scale N = 14	0.267 N.S.								
Q2-scale N = 15	2.249 p<.012	0.302 0.185	0.417 0.218	0.000 0.000	-0.262 0.262	0.372 0.225	1.118 0.181	0.407 0.261	0.145 0.260
Q3-scale N = 15	-0.844 N.S.								
Q4-scale N = 16	-3.378 p<.0004	-0.382 0.125	-0.334 0.133	-0.246 0.246	-0.219 0.128	-0.358 0.182	-0.831 0.210	-0.402 0.159	-0.349 0.223

b. EPI   Studies

Measure	Zst	Mn-ES	ES-m	ES-f	ES-ya	ES-ma	ES-ea	ES-sur	ES-exp
E-scale N = 12	-1.198 N.S.								
N-scale N = 12	-1.175 N.S.								

c. MMPI Studies

Measure	Zst	Mn-ES	ES-m	ES-f	ES-ya	ES-ma	ES-ea	ES-sur	ES-exp
Hs N = 7	-4.048 p<.00001	-0.518 0.125	-0.504 0.027	-- --	-0.558 --	-0.511 0.148	-- --	-0.620 0.130	-0.261 0.261
D N = 8	-4.975 p<.00001	-0.397 0.156	-0.576 0.121	-- --	-0.449 --	-0.389 0.180	-- --	-0.558 0.155	0.087 0.087

(table continues)

(Table 9.6, continued)

Measure	Zst	Mn-ES	ES-m	ES-f	ES-ya	ES-ma	ES-ea	ES-sur	ES-exp
Hy									
N = 7	-2.370	-0.133	-0.595	--	-0.558	-0.062	--	-0.221	0.087
	p<.0089	0.185	0.036	--	--	0.202	--	0.254	0.087
Pd									
N = 6	-1.384								
	N.S.								
Mf									
N = 6	-0.518								
	N.S.								
Pa									
N = 6	-1.453								
	N.S.								
Pt									
N = 6	-4.732	-0.599	-0.691	--	-1.148	-0.489	--	-0.719	0.000
	p<.00001	0.187	0.242	--	--	0.186	--	0.176	--
Sc									
N = 6	-2.707	-0.202	-0.515	--	-0.842	-0.074	--	-0.242	0.000
	p<.0034	0.170	0.185	--	--	0.137	--	0.202	--
Ma									
N = 6	1.057								
	N.S.								
Si									
N = 6	-3.327	-0.418	-0.420	--	-0.894	-0.323	--	-0.502	0.000
	p<.0004	0.215	0.242	--	--	0.237	--	0.243	--

EPI

1. Main effects.: As shown in Table 9.6b, mean changes on the E-scale (extraversion) and the N-scale (neuroticism) were both not significant. Therefore no further results of the meta-analysis of EPI data are reported.

MMPI

1. Main effects. As can be seen in Table 9.6c, 6 of the 10 MMPI scales showed significant effects: hypochondriasis ($Z = -4.048$), depression ($Z = -4.975$), hysteria ($Z = -2.370$), psychasthenia ($Z = -4.732$), schizophrenia ($Z = -2.707$), and social introversion ($Z = -3.327$). Mean scores on all scales decreased, as shown by the negative Z scores, and all of the decreases were significant at well beyond $p<.01$ and in the predicted direction. However, because of the small number of experiment studies in this group, some of these findings must regarded as tentative at present, a problem we address below.

2. Male-female differences. As is shown in Table 9.6c, all of the studies in the MMPI group were of male subjects, hence no gender comparisons are possible.

3. Age differences. All but one of the studies in the MMPI group were of middle-aged subjects, with the one exception being a group of young adults. Therefore, no conclusions about elderly groups can be made. In addition, while the noted decreases in hypochondriasis, depression, hysteria. psychasthenia, schizophrenia, and social introversion scores were observed in the one group of young adults, the decreases in hysteria and schizophrenia scores in the middle-aged groups were very close to zero. The decreases in hypochondriasis, depression, psychasthenia, and social introversion scores in the middle-aged groups, however, appeared to be reliable.

4. Survey versus experiment differences.: The reports in the MMPI group were, for all practical purposes, survey studies; therefore. any conclusions from the meta-analysis are tenuous. This problem may appear to be similar to that encountered in the EPI group, but there is at least

one important difference: the MMPI findings can be compared in part with those in earlier chapters, most notably
the mood, depression, and anxiety groups in chapters 6 and
7.   For example, our finding in Table 9.6c that the depression and psychasthenia scales showed the most significant decreases is in clear support of our similar findings
of decreases in tension and depression scores on the POMS,
and anxiety and depression scores on the MAACL in chapter
6, and measures of depression and anxiety in the depression
and anxiety groups in chapter 7.

The observed decreases on the remaining MMPI scales
(hypochondriasis, hysteria, schizophrenia, and social introversion) are not so easily compared with previous chapters
and must therefore await further validation.

5. *Clinical versus normal range studies.* One problem pe-
culiar to the MMPI group was that all but two were studies
of clinical groups, leaving only two normal range studies
(17P and 25P).   These studies, as did those noted above,
reported decreases in depression and psychasthenia scores.
In addition, both normal range studies reported decreases
in hypochondriasis and social introversion scores; however,
they were inconsistent on reported changes in hysteria and
schizophrenia scores, one reporting an increase and one
reporting a decrease.

The general finding in the MMPI group therefore seems
to be that there were (1) significant decreases in depression
and psychasthenia scores, highly consistent with our earlier
findings, (2) similar decreases in hypochondriasis and social
introversion scores, not as yet verified, and (3) inconsistent
decreases in hysteria and schizophrenia scores that may
not withstand further test.

Additional Comparisons

A summary of mean effects by method of calculation
of effect sizes for each of the personality inventories is
presented in Table 9.7.   As can be seen from the summary
in this table, there is little evidence to suggest that the
results described in this chapter were seriously affected
by method of calculating effect size.   The lone exception
would appear to be the studies in the 16PF group, where

Table 9.7. Additional data showing differences by method of
          calculating effect size.

	No. of studies	Mean effect size	Standard error
A. 16PF Group			
1. Full formula	3	-0.168	0.056
2. Glass formula	7	-0.014	0.171
3. Using t, F, etc.	5	-0.008	0.266
4. Using norm data	2	0.445	0.279
B. MMPI Group			
1. Full formula	0	--	--
2. Glass formula	5	-0.295	0.070
3. Using t, F, etc.	3	-0.564	0.144
4. Using norm data	0	--	--

Note: Effect sizes were calculated calculated by either (1) full
      formula, (2) Glass formula, (3) derived from another statistic,
      such as t, F, etc., or (4) by using norm data in place of
      absent controls.

normative data were used in place of a missing control group. Because there were only two studies where this was done, the net impact is not considered noteworthy.

As in previous chapters, we also attempted to compare studies by type of exercise to determine if there were differences in effect size, however, this proved to be impractical since nearly all of the studies in the personality group reported use of running/jogging as the primary form of exercise.

General Findings

The overall findings of the meta-analysis in the personality group may be summarized as follows:

1. The 16PF studies indicate significant effects on measures of intelligence (+), insecurity (-), self-sufficiency (+), and tension (-). The MMPI studies indicate significant effects on measures of depression (-) and psychasthenia (-), consistent with earlier findings, plus effects on measures of hypochondriasis (-) and social introversion (-) that require further verification, and tentative effects on measures of hysteria (-) and schizophrenia (-) that may prove difficult to verify.

2. Female groups were notably absent in the entire personality group, making all gender comparisons difficult or impossible.

3. Similarly, age comparisons in the personality group were difficult because of the narrow range represented, however, it was noted that there were few differences between young and middle-aged adults in the 16PF group. Elderly adults, however, showed greater effects on self-sufficiency (+) and tension (-) than the other age groups, plus effects on intelligence (-) and insecurity (+) that were the opposite of both younger groups. These results strongly suggest that there may be significant age differences in the effects of aerobic fitness training on measures of personality traits, some of which favor the elderly and some of which do not, clearly a tantalizing hypothesis for further study.

4. Differences between survey and experiment reports
    were not significant in the 16PF group, however,
    the absence of experiment reports did present a
    partial problem in the MMPI group. High corre-
    spondence with earlier results probably verifies the
    finding of a decrease in MMPI depression and psy-
    chasthenia scores, however, other MMPI findings
    must be regarded as tentative at this time. Both
    clinical and normal range groups demonstrated the
    decreases in MMPI depression and psychasthenia
    scores.
5. There were only minor differences as a function
    of method of calculating effect size. Nearly all
    of the studies in the personality group were studies
    of the effects of running/jogging exercise, so that
    no comparisons with other forms of exercise were
    possible.

Interpretation of Findings

Clearly the most interpretable findings in the personality group are the decreases in scores on insecurity and
tension, plus the increase in scores on self-sufficiency from
the 16PF. It requires no stretch of the imagination to
learn that individuals who complete an aerobic fitness
program describe themselves as less insecure and tense,
and more self-sufficient, along with the previously noted
improvements in mood and self-concept.

Of added interest, Noller et al. (1987) have shown that
16PF scores on insecurity and tension show a high positive
load on a factor labeled "emotional stability versus neuroticism" by Noller et al. and Digman and Inouye (1986) as
one of the "Big Five" robust factors of personality. Furthermore, scores on self-sufficiency load negatively on another of the five factors, termed social conformity or
agreeableness. Thus, it would appear that two of the five
factors show evidence of positive change as a result of
aerobic fitness training, that is, an increase in emotional
stability or a decrease in neuroticism, plus an increase in
self-sufficiency or a decrease in social conformity or
agreeableness.

The noted increase in intelligence on the 16PF does not appear to fit into this scheme as cleanly, although it does raise further possibilities.   To our knowledge, the 16PF B-scale is the only scale (from a personality inventory) that is based on the subject's ability to answer questions with a right or wrong answer. Our tentative interpretation of these results, therefore, is that the change in scores on intelligence reflect an improvement in cognitive function as a result of fitness training. Clearly, this is a hypothesis that would bear future investigation.   Some investigators (Clarkson-Smith and Hartley, 1989, 1990) have reported significant effects of exercise on cognitive functioning, whereas other investigators (Blumenthal and Madden, 1988; Madden, Blumenthal, Allen, and Emory, 1989) have failed to find such effects. Similarly, in a review of the research published through 1985, Tomporowski and Ellis (1986) concluded that the relationship between exercise and short-term facilitative effects on cognitive tasks is "problematic."   Because the resolution of this question could have enormous therapeutic consequences, we strongly urge that it be pursued vigorously.

Curiously, not one of the 16PF studies reported precisely the same effects identified by the meta-analysis. In fact, none was even close. Hence the meta-analysis clearly identified a unique combination of effects not previously reported.

Turning to another personality inventory, the results of the meta-analysis of the EPI data must be described as disappointing. There is little or no correspondence between the EPI data and all of the other findings, and we see little reason to support the use of the EPI in future studies of the effects of aerobic fitness training at this time.

In contrast, although the results of the meta-analysis of the MMPI data may be taken as tentative, we do not find them discouraging. Indeed, the finding of decreased scores on the depression and psychasthenia scales is highly interpretable and consistent with an array of reasonably clear-cut data.   Other noted decreases in scores on hypochondriasis and social introversion scales also merit further investigation. Undoubtedly, there is a strong need in this group for more studies of normal subjects. The frequently heard belief that the MMPI is only suitable for studies of clinical groups is probably exaggerated and leads to some missed opportunity to expand our insights in a complex area.

Another problem that should be examined again is the consequence of having to conduct a meta-analysis for each scale for each of the personality inventories, which resulted in a total of 28 separate meta-analyses, and in turn raised the prospect of a Type I error. That is, one would expect at least one significant effect at $p<.05$ by chance alone in a group of 28 comparisons. We note, however, that all of the significant effects in the 16PF and MMPI groups were beyond $p<.02$, and in most cases well beyond $p<.01$. The likelihood of a Type I error in these findings therefore does not seem compelling.

Lastly, although it is tempting to suggest that the overall findings in the meta-analysis in the personality group indicate that aerobic fitness training produces relatively enduring changes in personality traits as measured by objective personality inventories, such a conclusion is still premature. Until such time as long-term follow-up data are routinely included, conclusions about the duration of *any* changes produced by aerobic fitness training are unwarranted. This is not to say that the data thus far are not encouraging -- indeed they are highly so -- suggesting that' the missing steps (long-term follow-up observations) are all the more imperative. On an a priori basis, we might anticipate that changes reflected in the 16PF, consistent with the notion of five robust personality factors, should stand the best chances of demonstrating some enduring characteristics, whereas the noted changes in MMPI depression and psychasthenia scores might be more likely to be sensitive to transient shifts akin to mood scores. Further work on these intriguing hypotheses should not be difficult.

Summary

In this chapter, we present the results of a meta-analysis of studies of the effects of aerobic fitness training on measures of personality, which be summarized as follows:

1. Personality, as used in this context, is measured solely by objective personality questionnaires that are based on a trait-defined view of personality. These traits are usually defined as relatively enduring characteristics, in contrast to transient measures, such as mood state.

2. Nine different personality inventories were represented in studies found on this topic. However, only three inventories were represented in sufficient number to support a meta-analysis: the 16PF, EPI, and MMPI. Because the trait measures generated by each questionnaire are often nonoverlapping, it was necessary to conduct a meta-analysis for each scale for each inventory.

3. Thirty-one studies comprised the personality group. For each study, the following information was given: subject group(s), number of males and females per group, mean age, experimental design, type of effect size, and measure of fitness.

4. The results of the meta-analyses were presented for each scale for each inventory, including main effects, gender differences, age differences, survey versus experiment differences, and differences by method of calculating effect sizes.

5. Significant effects in the 16PF group were increases in measures of intelligence and self-sufficiency and decreases in measures of insecurity and tension. None of the individual 16PF studies reported precisely the same unique combination of effects identified by the meta-analysis. Effects in the MMPI group were decreases in scores on hypochondriasis, depression, hysteria, psychasthenia, schizophrenia, and social introversion. The EPI findings were not statistically significant.

6. Decreases in 16PF measures of insecurity and tension suggest a corresponding change in one of five robust factors, that is, emotional stability versus neuroticism. Similarly, increases in the 16PF measure of self-sufficiency suggest a decrease in another of the five robust factors, namely, social conformity or agreeableness. The MMPI findings of decreased scores on depression and psychasthenia

fit well with the mood, depression, and anxiety data presented in previous chapters.

7.   The increases in scores on intelligence on the 16PF suggest some improvement in cognitive function that would merit further study.

8.   Several gaps in the reported studies were noted. Most troublesome were: (1) the lack of experiment studies in both the EPI and MMPI groups, (2) the relative lack of female groups in the personality group as a whole, (3) the preponderance of middle-aged groups to the underrepresentation of young and elderly adults, (4) the lack of normal groups in the MMPI studies, and (5) the total lack, throughout every chapter of this book, of long-term follow-up data.

9.   Several areas of future effort were vigorously recommended.

TEN

THEORY AND CONCLUSIONS

This chapter consists of three parts: (1) a summary of the findings reported in chapters 6 through 9, (2) discussion of a theoretical model of the psychological effects of aerobic fitness training, based in part on previously published theoretical work and in part on the results of our meta-analysis, and (3) indicated directions for future research.

Summary of Results

Because this book is a review of the psychological effects of aerobic fitness training, using the quantitative method of meta-analysis, an attempt was made to identify all pertinent studies. The final group comprised a total of 90 studies that appeared through 1988, although some more recent studies were found and included, with subgroups as follows: mood group (26 studies), depression group (15 studies), anxiety group (22 studies), self-concept group (37 studies, and personality group (31 studies). This is a total of 131 studies, however, some of them appeared in more than one group.

We begin with a summary of the most significant results of the meta-analyses of previous chapters. Obviously, this presents an opportunity to bring together a large number of observations for a new and potentially far-reaching perspective.

Main Effects

The significant main effects from each of the previous chapters are given in descending rank order of effect size in Table 10.1. Such a rank-ordering provides information on the question of "What effects are significant?" and potentially more important "What are the largest effects?"

Several interpretations of the data summarized in Table 10.1 appear to be warranted. For example, measures that presumably assess the same (or related aspects of) one

Table 10.1. Mean effect sizes and standard error of all significant main effects in descending rank order, disregarding sign.

Measure-Test	Effect Size	S.E.
Depression--MAACL	-1.120	0.343
Anxiety--MAACL	-0.988	0.218
Depression--mixed tests	-0.967	0.182
Psychasthenia--MMPI	-0.599	0.187
Self-concept--mixed tests	0.560	0.087
Hypochondriasis--MMPI	-0.518	0.125
Social introversion--MMPI	-0.418	0.215
Confusion--POMS	-0.402	0.075
Vigor--POMS	0.399	0.077
Depression--MMPI	-0.397	0.156
Q4 (tension)--16PF	-0.382	0.125
B (intelligence)--16PF	0.378	0.152
Tension--POMS	-0.322	0.060
Q2 (self-sufficiency)--16PF	0.302	0.185
Depression--POMS	-0.284	0.068
Anxiety-state--STAI	-0.279	0.095
Fatigue--POMS	-0.271	0.062
Anxiety-trait--STAI	-0.254	0.070
Schizophrenia--MMPI	-0.202	0.170
O (insecurity)--16PF	-0.185	0.112
Hysteria--MMPI	-0.133	0.185

concept may be grouped or clustered on a rational basis. We have identified four such clusters, three of which are highly supportable at this time. In decreasing order of mean effect size, the four clusters are the depression cluster, the anxiety cluster, the self-concept cluster, and the adjustment cluster.

Depression Cluster. This group consists of seven effects of the 21 listed in Table 10.1. In decreasing rank order the group consists of:

1. Depression -- MAACL (-)
2. Depression -- mixed tests (-)
3. Confusion -- POMS (-)
4. Vigor -- POMS (+)
5. Depression -- MMPI (-)
6. Depression -- POMS (-)
7. Fatigue -- POMS (-)

The mean effect size (disregarding sign) of this group was 0.549, and the standard error (SE) was 0.131. The POMS confusion, vigor, and fatigue scores were included in the depression cluster because of the reported correlation between these scores and POMS depression scores (McNair, Lorr & Droppleman, 1971, p. 9).

As indicated in chapter 7, these results are likely a reflection of the effects of aerobic fitness training, rather than an effect of extraneous variables. There is probably some expectancy (or other confound) effect in the MAACL depression scores, however, the case for this interpretation is not persuasive for the other measures in the depression cluster. This does not establish the nature of a causal relationship, nor does it suggest that fitness training is any more than one of a number of possible therapeutic approaches in dealing with depression. However, it does indicate that aerobic fitness training is associated with significant improvement in measures of depression.

Anxiety Cluster. This group consists of six effects of those listed in Table 10.1. In decreasing order, the group includes (all as decreases):

1. Anxiety -- MAACL

2. Psychasthenia -- MMPI
3. Q4 (tension) -- 16PF
4. Tension -- POMS
5. Anxiety-State -- STAI
6. Anxiety-Trait -- STAI

The mean effect size for the group was 0.471 (SE = 0.115). Here too, it is our view that these results are a reflection of the effects of aerobic fitness training, rather than a confound effect, with the sole likely exception of the MAACL anxiety scores.

Self-Esteem Cluster. This group includes three measures:

1. Self-concept -- mixed tests (+)
2. Q2 (self-sufficiency) -- 16PF (+)
3. O (insecurity) -- 16PF (-)

The mean effect size was 0.349 (SE = 0.111). The consistency of this finding, especially in the case of mixed tests (based on all of the data reported in chapter 8), is an essential component of the theoretical model presented later in this chapter. In addition, because of the relatively large number of inventories and studies included in this cluster, we have chosen the global concept of self-esteem as a more appropriate identifier over self-concept. Concerns about confound effects in these studies have not been as notable as with studies of depression and anxiety.

Adjustment Cluster. This group consists of five measures (four from the MMPI and one from the 16PF) that may eventually prove to be more than one group. It was noted in chapter 9 that the MMPI measures in this cluster were derived largely from survey, rather than experiment, studies. Consequently it must still be regarded as tentative, especially since there is as yet no independent verification, unlike that noted for the findings reported for the MMPI depression and psychasthenia scales. The adjustment cluster includes:

1. Hypochondriasis -- MMPI (-)
2. Social introversion -- MMPI (-)
3. Intelligence -- 16PF (+)

4.   Schizophrenia -- MMPI (-)
5.   Hysteria -- MMPI (-)

The mean effect size was 0.330 (SE = 0.071).

Male-Female Differences
   In general, it was shown that males and females demonstrated highly similar, but not identical overall effects
across all measures in the meta-analysis. Male groups did
indeed show all of the listed main effects, and, although
the female groups did not quite show all of the same effects, the gender differences do not appear to be major.
Female groups showed the same self-concept effects and
most of the mood effects, although there were two cases
where female groups did not show a mood effect observed
in males, specifically, females did not show the decreases
in MAACL-depression and both the state and trait scores
of the STAI. Finally, female groups were notably absent
from the personality group, making gender comparisons
impossible in this instance. We would thus conclude that
there is little or no evidence of significant gender differences, although it would obviously be wise if investigators
included more female groups in future studies, especially
those directed at personality effects.

Age Differences
   All of the main effects listed in Table 10.1 were observed in young adults (<30) and middle-aged adults (30-60).
However, there were inconsistencies (and very large gaps)
in the results for elderly adults (>60). That is, elderly adult
groups showed all of the effects on self-concept and depression shown by the younger groups, but not the effect
on anxiety. Of course there were not many elderly groups
in each of these meta-analyses. Furthermore, there were
no demonstrated effects on mood and inconsistent effects
on personality measures in elderly groups, primarily because
elderly subjects were seriously underrepresented in these
meta-analyses. Therefore, the biggest single age finding
in these analyses is that very few elderly groups have been
studied to date, making confident conclusions impossible
at this time. It is encouraging to note that, where elderly
subjects have been included, the observed effects are almost the same as in younger groups, although not identical

-- a finding that raises intriguing, but as yet unanswered, questions.

Survey versus Experiment Differences

Survey versus experiment comparisons were made as a part of each meta-analysis in order to assess the effects of experimental rigor. It was heartening therefore to find that there were no systematic differences in effect sizes between survey and experiment reports, with two exceptions. As noted previously, the POMS anger effects were not significant in the experiment studies (although they were so in the survey studies), and thus the POMS anger results were not included in Table 10.1. In addition, there was the problem that there were almost no experiment studies in the MMPI group, leaving much of these results inconclusive.

Method of Calculating Effect Size

There were no systematic effects on the results of the meta-analyses as a result of the method of calculating effect sizes. Four different methods of calculation were available, and the choice depended on the completeness of reporting in the original article.

Type of Exercise

We had originally planned to make some statements about the effects of different types of exercise. However, we found that the choices are too narrow to support any clear-cut conclusion. An overwhelming majority of the studies were limited to running/jogging/walking as the form of exercise, and therefore our results and conclusions apply primarily to aerobic fitness achieved in this manner. Although we have no compelling reason to suspect that other forms of exercise are more effective, there remains some possibility that different forms of exercise may elicit differences in speed or efficiency of effects or in long-term impact.

Additional Conclusions

It should be noted that some additional conclusions were reached in the individual preceding chapters, for example, on the choice of measure for those variables (such as depression or self-concept) for which several are available.

The reader is referred to specific chapters for information about these questions.

Theoretical Models

Given the wealth of demonstrated findings on the psychological effects of aerobic fitness training, we now turn to the task of considering the most appropriate theoretical model. We acknowledge that fitness training also produces a host of physiological, biochemical, metabolic and other effects (e.g., see Morgan, 1985; Morgan & Goldston, 1987; Williams & Wallace, 1989); however, consideration of processes at these levels is beyond the scope of this book.

Sonstroem Model

A major theoretical contribution that has received sustained attention is the psychological model for physical activity proposed by Sonstroem (1978). His fundamental notion was that physical exercise, and the resulting physical fitness, leads to increased estimation of physical abilities (physical self-concept) as part of total self-esteem, which in turn leads to increased attraction to (interest in) physical exercise, and so on in a repetitive loop. This model was originally demonstrated by Sonstroem in adolescent males in a correlational study based largely on the PEAS (which Sonstroem developed). Dishman (1978) and Fox, Corbin, and Couldry (1985) later demonstrated the effectiveness of Sonstroem's model with undergraduates, and McDonald, Norton, and Hodgdon (1990), and McDonald, Beckett, and Hodgdon (1991) obtained similar results with military groups.

The success of this model is also due to additional features, including (a) its fit with general intuitive beliefs about the mediating effects of psychological constructs on physical fitness measures, (b) that the author assigned "self-esteem" as the ultimate or highest hierarchical end-product of physical fitness training, a view supported and documented in great detail by Sonstroem (1984) and by Fox and Corbin (1989), and (c) that each of the constructs within the model is operationally defined by instruments of some genuine utility. For example, in addition to Sonstroem's original data, Safrit, Wood, and Dishman (1985) found that the PEAS demonstrates several measurable strengths, although some items could be cut to shorten the total scale.

At the same time, the model as originally proposed was described by Sonstroem (1978, 1984) as tentative at best, suggesting that some refinements would eventually be required. For example, any model based on a repetitive loop of effects must eventually be validated with longitudinal data, a missing element in Sonstroem's original report. In addition, the measurement devices for some of his constructs were in need of improvement, for example, global self-esteem measures as discussed by Fox and Corbin. Thus Sonstroem and Morgan (1989) introduced a notable revision over the original model. The primary modifications in the revised model are:

1. Longitudinal data. Clear emphasis is placed on the need for repeated or serial measures for periods up to 1 to 2 years to establish the longitudinal relationships between exercise and self-esteem more firmly.
2. Continuum of self-perceptions. Self-perceptions are placed on a continuum in the model from the most specific (physical self-efficacy) to the most general (self-esteem).
3. Improved measurement. Stress is given to the need for experimentation in development of construct measures, such as physical competence (especially in middle-aged groups) and global self-esteem.

Other major features of the original model are retained by Sonstroem and Morgan, namely, the repetitive loop of exercise effects on self-esteem, as well as the notion that adjacent constructs within the model are more highly correlated than constructs separated by or more steps on the specific-to-general continuum of self-perceptions.

McDonald-Manley Model
In addition to the considerations given by Sonstroem (1978) and Sonstroem and Morgan (1989), there is an undeniable body of evidence demonstrating that a number of additional variables serve as mediators in the effect of exercise and fitness on self-esteem.

Dishman (1978, 1982, 1984; Dishman & Ickes, 1981; Dishman, Ickes & Morgan, 1980) has shown overwhelmingly that motivational considerations serve as highly significant mediators in exercise adherence. This is a view supported by McDonald, et al. (1991), and by Hogan (1989), as well as numerous others.

Furthermore, the results of the meta-analysis clearly demonstrate that mood (i.e., depression and anxiety) and adjustment variables serve as significant mediators between fitness and self-esteem, plus the added conclusion that self-esteem itself is significantly enhanced by fitness training. For these reasons, McDonald and Manley (1991) proposed a general model of the role of mediators in the effects of exercise and fitness on self-esteem, illustrated in Figure 1. This model presupposes an interactive relationship between the general class of mediators and self-esteem. In addition, since a repetitive loop is mathematically awkward as a means of describing longitudinal effects, we depict the processes serially by means of the labels "Time 1," "Time 2," and "Time 3." Thus, the model postulates effects over time and therefore requires longitudinal data for ultimate validation.

As noted in Figure 1, the general mediator class undoubtedly includes an indeterminant number of intervening variables, such as mood, adjustment, motivation, physical self-concept, and interests. The precise nature of the interactive relationship between each of these mediating variables is a project that would require both longitudinal data and significant elaboration of the mediator component of the general model, potentially a highly fruitful challenge for future research.

Structural Equation Modeling

In a parallel set of developments, in recent years there have been remarkable improvements in technical methods and capacity for model building. For example, impressive techniques now exist for developing theoretical models involving latent (or unobserved theoretical) variables, using sophisticated software packages for path analysis and structural equation modeling (Anderson & Gerbing, 1988; Bentler & Bonett, 1980; Loehlin, 1987). Although this relatively new statistical method has not yet been applied to the Sonstroem model, Clarkson-Smith and Hartley (1990)

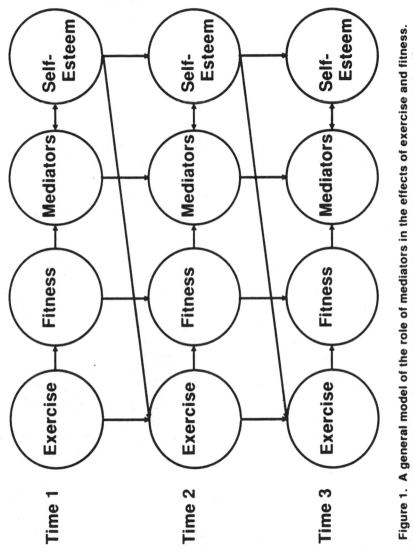

Figure 1. A general model of the role of mediators in the effects of exercise and fitness. "Mediators" includes a number of variables, such as mood, motivation, physical self-concept, interest in exercise, and others. Time 1, Time 2, and Time 3 depict longitudinal effects.

have shown that structural equation models of the relationships between exercise and cognitive performance in
an elderly group fit the data well.   They acknowledge that
longitudinal data are still necessary to establish a causal
relationship more firmly; however, the structural equation
model does add significant evidence that exercise promotes
cognitive processing in the elderly.   This result clearly
warrants more long-term study.

Guidelines for Future Research

As a final topic, but not the last in importance by any
criterion, we turn our attention to a consideration of recommended guidelines and directions for future research.
After an extended exposure to the literature in this field,
we believe that much is still clearly needed, just as some
other research is no longer urgent.

Choice of Subject Groups

Of all subject groups, the greatest need is for studies
of the elderly, both male and female, employing forms of
exercise more suitable for the elderly than running/jogging,
such as walking, swimming, or bike riding.   Absence of
valuable knowledge here could work a serious (but avoid-
able) hardship on society in the coming decades.   For example, there are tantalizing suggestions in the existing data
that fitness training might have a protective (if not a
therapeutic) effect on cognitive functioning in the elderly,
although numerous questions remain.   If such a protective
effect can be demonstrated with rigorous longitudinal data,
the long-range potential benefits for society could be
enormous.

Similarly, there is need for additional studies of female
groups of all ages.   Young adult male groups are probably
the least needed, but even this most common group was
underrepresented (as were young adult females) in the
studies of personality effects with the MMPI.

Lastly, there is little general need for additional studies
of effects on depression, except in male or female elderly
groups.   Since the incidence of depression increases in the
elderly, the therapeutic potential of fitness training for this
group should be fully exploited.   Additional studies of other

patient groups, such as anxiety-prone or coronary-risk subjects, could be highly valuable.

What Effects to Study?

As stated repeatedly in this book, there is an undeniable
need for further rigorous study of the effects of fitness
training on cognitive functioning and on personality trait
measures, whereas there is almost no remaining need to
study effects on mood or self-concept, except in the elderly.

Both cognitive functioning and personality traits are
relatively generic labels for categories of behavior that
include a nonspecific number of functions and characteristics, and therefore the need to disentangle these processes
in significant. Investigators must choose their measures
with great care, because the cost of a poor choice could
be great.

For example, many answers about personality effects
are muddled, because too many investigators have relied
on personality inventories of marginal utility. We strongly
recommend greater use of second- or third-generation instruments, such as the NEO Personality Inventory (Costa
& McCrae, 1985) and the Physical Self-Perception Profile
(Fox & Corbin, 1989), two instruments that could be used
to advantage in future studies. Doubtless there are other
newly introduced instruments that could be equally well
suited.

Experimental Design

Of all considerations in designing future studies, perhaps
none is more important than the need to include longitudinal and follow-up data, in all age, gender, and patient
groups studied. Firmly established theory and most practical applications of the major findings will necessarily be
delayed until this void is eliminated.

We also strongly encourage more experiment (as opposed
to survey) studies, with random assignment to groups
wherever possible, and pre- and posttest measurements.
It was reassuring to find that there were no systematic
differences between survey and experiment studies. Nevertheless, the question of the effects on depression was
not answered until there were sufficient numbers of well-
controlled experiment studies, and the confound interpre-

tation could be reasonably ruled out. We especially applaud the increased attention to controls for subject biasing effects, most notably expectancy effects, plus regression effects and spontaneous remission in clinical groups.

More Thorough Reporting

The completeness of the reporting is spotty, and at times appalling. Subjects should always be fully described, including the number of males and females, mean ages for both (if appropriate), means and standard deviations of both pre- and posttest observations. Results of the statistical analysis, whether statistically significant or not, should be specified clearly.

Refinement of Theory

As a final step, additional work on theory, both development and validation, is needed. We do not propose a proliferation of model building, however, there is a clear need for longitudinal data in support of existing models, plus more refined measurement of theoretical constructs comprising these models. New techniques, such as structural equation modeling, would appear to hold significant promise. A number of phenomena are clearly established as mediating variables in the effects of exercise and fitness on self-esteem, but the precise nature of their interactive relationship is in need of much further work.

The fact that aerobic fitness training produces a number of significant psychological effects is now well established, and the opportunity to enlarge on these findings represents a truly exciting and highly valuable contribution for years to come. A meaningful improvement in the human condition should be accomplished as a result.

APPENDIX A

Statistical Formulae

Statistical formulae for the meta-analysis:

$$ES = \frac{(M_{E_2} - M_{E_1}) - (M_{C_2} - M_{C_1})}{S_{(E_1 + C_1)}} \qquad (1)$$

$$S^2_{(E_1 + C_1)} = \frac{(N_E - 1)(S_{E_1})^2 + (N_C - 1)(S_{C_1})^2}{N_E + N_C - 2} \qquad (2)$$

$$K = 1 - \frac{3}{4(N_E + N_C - 2) - 1} \qquad (3)$$

Where:

ES = effect size
E = experimental group
C = control group
M = mean
S = standard deviation
1 = pretest
2 = posttest
K = correction

Coding Summary

The following is a reproduction (somewhat reduced) of the coding sheet used to summarize information about each study prior to the meta-analysis.

Test group(s):_____

Author(s):_____

Title:_____
_____

Journal:_____
_____Year_____Vol_____Pgs_____

Experimental Design_____
Measure of fitness_____
Fitness training protocol_____
Independent variable(s)_____
   Group 1 name_____   Group 2 name_____
   Sex #M_____ #F_____   Sex #M_____ #F_____
   Age(mn & range)_____   Age(mn & range)_____

Dependent variable(s):

   Measure #1_____
   Pretest Mean_____sd_____   Mean_____sd_____
   Posttest Mean_____sd_____   Mean_____sd_____
            Test_____df error_____
            Test value_____Z_____
            p-level_____effect size_____

   Measure #2_____
   Pretest Mean_____sd_____   Mean_____sd_____
   Posttest Mean_____sd_____   Mean_____sd_____
            Test_____df error_____
            Test value_____Z_____
            p-level_____effect size_____

   Measure #3_____
   Pretest Mean_____sd_____   Mean_____sd_____
   Posttest Mean_____sd_____   Mean_____sd_____
            Test_____df error_____
            Test value_____Z_____
            p-level_____effect size_____

2

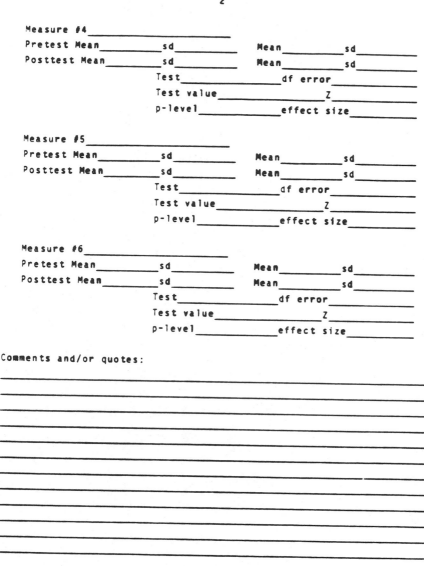

Measure #4_____

Pretest Mean_____ sd_____   Mean_____ sd_____

Posttest Mean_____ sd_____   Mean_____ sd_____

                    Test_____ df error_____

                    Test value_____ Z_____

                    p-level_____ effect size_____

Measure #5_____

Pretest Mean_____ sd_____   Mean_____ sd_____

Posttest Mean_____ sd_____   Mean_____ sd_____

                    Test_____ df error_____

                    Test value_____ Z_____

                    p-level_____ effect size_____

Measure #6_____

Pretest Mean_____ sd_____   Mean_____ sd_____

Posttest Mean_____ sd_____   Mean_____ sd_____

                    Test_____ df error_____

                    Test value_____ Z_____

                    p-level_____ effect size_____

Comments and/or quotes:

_____
_____
_____
_____
_____
_____
_____
_____
_____
_____
_____
_____
_____
_____

REFERENCES

Abadie, B. R. (1988). Relating trait anxiety to perceived physical fitness. *Perceptual and Motor Skills,* 67, 539-543.

Abelson, P. H. (1968). Physical fitness. *Science, 161,* 1299.

Aloia, J. F., Cohn, S. H., Ostuni, J. A., Cane, R., & Ellis, K. (1978). Prevention of involutional bone loss by exercise. *Annals of Internal Medicine, 89,* 356-358.

American College of Sports Medicine. (1978). The recommended quantity and quality of exercise for developing and maintaining fitness in healthy adults. *Medicine and Science in Sports,* 10, vii-x.

American College of Sports Medicine. (1984). Prevention of injuries during distance running. *Medicine and Science in Sports and Exercise, 16,* ix-xiv.

American College of Sports Medicine. (1991). *Guidelines for Exercise Testing and Prescription* (4th ed.). Philadelphia: Lea & Febiger.

Anastasi, A. (1982). *Psychological Testing* (5th ed.). New York: Macmillan.

Anderson, J. C., & Gerbing, D. W. (1988). Structural equation modeling in practice: A review and recommended two-step approach. *Psychological Bulletin, 103,* 411-423.

Baekeland, F., & Lasky, R. (1966). Exercise and sleep patterns in college athletes. *Perceptual and Motor Skills,* 23, 1203-1207.

Bangert-Drowns, R. L. (1986). Review of developments in meta-analytic method. *Psychological Bulletin, 99,* 388-399.

Bassler, T., and Scaff, J. (1974). [Letter to the Editor] *New England Journal of Medicine, 291,* 1192.

Bassler, T., and Scaff, J. (1975). [Letter to the Editor] *New England Journal of Medicine, 292,* 1302.

Beck, A. T. (1967). *Depression: Clinical, Experimental, and Theoretical Aspects.* New York: Harper & Row.

Benjamin, L. S. (1974). Structural analysis of social behavior. *Psychological Review, 81,* 392-425.

Bentler, P. M. (1972). The Tennessee Self Concept Scale. In O. K. Buros (Ed.), *The seventh mental measurements yearbook* (pp. 366-367). Highland Park, NJ: Gryphon Press.

Bentler, P. M., & Bonett, D. G. (1980). Significance tests and goodness of fit in the analysis of covariance structures. *Psychological Bulletin, 88,* 588-606.

Ben-Shlomo, L. S., & Short, M. A. (1983). The effects of physical exercise on self-attitudes. *Occupational Therapy in Mental Health, 3,* 11-28.

Berger, B. G., & Owen, D. R. (1983). Mood alteration with swimming - swimmers really do "feel better." *Psychosomatic Medicine, 45*, 425-433.

Bills, R. E., Vance, E. L., & McLean, O. S. (1951). An index of adjustment and values. *Journal of Consulting Psychology, 15*, 257-261.

Blackman, L., Hunter, G., Hilyer, J., & Harrison, P. (1988). The effects of dance team participation on female adolescent physical fitness and self-concept. *Adolescence, 23*, 439-448.

Blair, S. N. (1984). How to assess exercise habits and physical fitness. In J. D. Matarazzo, S. M. Weiss, J. A. Herd, N. E. Miller, & S. M. Weiss (Eds.), *Behavioral health: A handbook of health enhancement and disease prevention* (pp. 424-447). New York: John Wiley.

Blair, S. N., Jacob, D. R., & Powell, K. E. (1985). Relationships between exercise or physical activity and other health behaviors. *Public Health Reports, 100*, 172-180.

Block, J. (1978). The Eysenck Personality Questionnaire. In O. K. Buros (Ed.), *The eighth mental measurements yearbook* (pp. 805-809). Highland Park, NJ: Gryphon Press.

Blomqvist, C. G., & Saltin, B. (1983). Cardiovascular adaptations to physical training. *Annual Review of Physiology, 45*, 169-189.

Bloxom, B. M. (1978). The 16PF Questionnaire. In O. K. Buros (Ed.), *The eighth mental measurements yearbook* (pp. 1077-1078). Highland Park, NJ: Gryphon Press.

Blumenthal, J. A., Emery, C. F., Madden, D. J., George, L. K., Coleman, R. E., Riddle, M. W., McKee, D. C., Reasoner, J., & Williams, R. S. (1989). Cardiovascular and behavioral effects of aerobic exercise training in healthy older men and women. *Journal of Gerontology, 44*, M147-M157.

Blumenthal, J. A., & Madden, D. J. (1988). Effects of aerobic exercise training, age, and physical fitness on memory-search performance. *Psychology and Aging, 3*, 280-285.

Blumenthal, J. A., Schocken, D. D., Needels, T. L., & Hindle, P. (1982). Psychological and physiological effects of physical conditioning on the elderly. *Journal of Psychosomatic Research, 26*, 505-510.

Blumenthal, J. A., Williams, R. S., Needels, T. L., & Wallace, A. G. (1982). Psychological changes accompany aerobic exercise in healthy middle-aged adults. *Psychosomatic Medicine, 44*, 529-536.

Bolton, B. F. (1978). The 16PF Questionnaire. In O. K. Buros (Ed.), *The eighth mental measurements yearbook* (pp. 1078-1080). Highland Park, NJ: Gryphon Press.

Bolton, B., & Milligan, T. (1976). The effects of a systematic physical fitness program on clients in a comprehensive rehabilitation center. *American Correctional Therapy Journal, 30*, 41-46.

Bonanno, J. A. (1977). Coronary risk factor modification by chronic physical exercise. In E. A. Amsterdam, J. H. Wilmore, & A. N. DeMaria (Eds.), *Exercise in cardiovascular health and disease* (pp. 274-279). New York: York Medical Books.

Bonanno, J. A., & Lies, J. E. (1974). Effect of physical training on coronary risk factors. *American Journal of Cardiology, 33,* 760-764.

Bowen, O. R. (1985). *Health, United States, 1985.* (DHHS Publication No. 86-1232.) Washington, DC: U.S. Government Printing Office.

Brinkman, J. R., & Hoskins, T. A. (1979). Physical conditioning and altered self-concept in rehabilitated hemiplegic patients. *Physical Therapy, 59,* 859-865.

Brown, E. Y., Morrow, J. R., Jr., & Livingston, S. M. (1982). Self-concept changes in women as a result of training. *Journal of Sport Psychology, 4,* 354-363.

Brown, R. S., Ramirez, D. E., & Taub, J. M. (1978). The prescription of exercise for depression. *The Physician and Sportsmedicine, 6,* 34, 36-37, 40-41, 44-45.

Browne, M. A., & Mahoney, M. J. (1984). Sport psychology. *Annual Review of Psychology, 35,* 605-625.

Buccola, V. A., & Stone, W. J. (1975). Effects of jogging and cycling programs on physiological and personality variables in aged men. *Research Quarterly, 46,* 134-139.

Buffone, G. W. (1984). Running and depression. In M. L. Sachs & G. W. Buffone (Eds.), *Running as therapy: An integrated approach* (pp. 6-22). Lincoln, NE: University of Nebraska Press.

Bullock, R. J., & Svyantek, D. J. (1985). Analyzing meta-analysis: Potential problems, an unsuccessful replication, and evaluation criteria. *Journal of Applied Psychology, 70,* 108-115.

Bunnell, D. E., Bevier, W., & Horvath, S. M. (1983). Effects of exhaustive exercise on the sleep of men and women. *Psychophysiology, 20,* 50-58.

Butcher, J. N. (1985). The 16PF Questionnaire. In J. V. Mitchell, Jr. (Ed.), *The ninth mental measurements yearbook* (pp. 1391-1392). Lincoln, NE: University of Nebraska Press.

Califano, J. A. (1979). *Healthy people: The Surgeon General's report on health promotion and disease prevention.* (DHEW Publication No. 79-55071.) Washington, DC: U.S. Government Printing Office.

Campbell, D. T. (1969). Reforms as experiments. *American Psychologist, 24,* 409-429.

Campbell, D. T., & Stanley, J. C. (1966). *Experimental and quasi-experimental designs for research.* Chicago: Rand McNally.

Cantwell, J. D. (1985). Cardiovascular aspects of running. *Clinics in Sports Medicine, 4,* 627-640.

Carney, R. M., McKevitt, P. M., Goldberg, A. P., Hagberg, J., Delmez, J. A., & Harter, H. R. (1983). Psychological effects of exercise training in hemodialysis patients. *Nephron, 33,* 179-181.

Cattell, R. B., Eber, H. W., & Tatsuoka, M. M. (1970). *Handbook of the 16PF Questionnaire.* Champaign, IL: Institute of Personality and Ability Testing.

Clarkson-Smith, L., & Hartley, A. A. (1989). Relationships between physical exercise and cognitive abilities in older adults. *Psychology and Aging, 4,* 183-189.

Clarkson-Smith, L., & Hartley, A. A. (1990). Structural equation models of relationships between exercise and cognitive abilities. *Psychology and Aging, 5,* 437-446.

Clausen, J. P. (1977). Effect of physical training on cardiovascular adjustments to exercise in man. *Physiological Reviews, 57*, 779-815.

Collingwood, T. R. (1972). The effects of physical training upon behavior and self attitudes. *Journal of Clinical Psychology, 28*, 583-585.

Collingwood, T. R., & Willett, L. (1971). The effects of physical training upon self-concept and body attitude. *Journal of Clinical Psychology, 27*, 411-412.

Contrada, R. J., Wright, R. A., & Glass, D. C. (1985). Psychophysiologic correlates of type A behavior: Comments on Houston (1983) and Holmes (1983). *Journal of Research in Personality, 19*, 12-30.

Cooper, H. M. (1989). *Integrating research: A guide for literature reviews* (2nd ed.). Beverly Hills, CA: Sage.

Cooper, H. M., & Rosenthal, R. (1980). Statistical versus traditional procedures for summarizing research findings. *Psychological Bulletin, 87*, 442-449.

Cooper, K. H. (1968). *Aerobics.* New York: Evans.

Cooper, K. H. (1970). *The new aerobics.* New York: Evans.

Cooper, K. H. (1977). *The aerobics way.* New York: Evans.

Cooper, K. H. (1982). *The aerobics program for total well-being.* New York: Evans.

Cooper, K. H. (1985). *Running without fear.* New York: Evans.

Cooper, K. H. (1988). *Controlling cholesterol: Dr. Kenneth H. Cooper's preventive medicine program.* New York: Bantam Books.

Cooper, K. H., Pollock, M. L., Martin, R. P., White, S. R., Linnerud, A. C., & Jackson, A. (1976). Physical fitness levels vs selected coronary risk factors: A cross-sectional study. *Journal of the American Medical Association, 236*, 166-169.

Cooper, M., & Cooper, K. H. (1972). *Aerobics for women.* New York: Evans.

Coopersmith, S. (1967). *The antecedents of self-esteem.* San Francisco: Freeman.

Coopersmith, S. (1981). *Self-esteem inventories.* Palo Alto, CA: Consulting Psychologists Press.

Costa, P. R. & McCrae, R. T. (1985). *Manual for the NEO Personality Inventory.* Baltimore: Psychological Assessment Resources, Inc.

Cureton, T. K. (1963). Improvement of psychological states by means of exercise-fitness programs. *Journal of the Association for Physical and Mental Rehabilitation, 17*, 14-17, 25.

Dahlstrom, W. G., Welsh, G. S., & Dahlstrom, L. E. (1972-1975). *An MMPI handbook* (rev. ed.). Minneapolis: University of Minnesota Press.

Derogatis, L. R., Lipman, R. S., & Covi, L. (1973). The SCL-90: An outpatient psychiatric rating scale. *Psychopharmacology Bulletin, 9*, 13-28.

Derogatis, L. R., Rickels, K., & Rock, A. F. (1976). The SCL-90 and the MMPI: A step in the validation of a new self-report scale. *British Journal of Psychiatry, 128*, 280-289.

Dienstbier, R. A. (1984). The effect of exercise on personality. In M. L. Sachs & G. W. Buffone (Eds.), *Running as therapy: An integrated approach* (pp. 253-272). Lincoln, NE: University of Nebraska Press.

Digman, J. M., & Inouye, J. (1986). Further specification of the five robust factors of personality. *Journal of Personality and Social Psychology, 50,* 116-123.

Digman, J. M., & Takemoto-Chock, N. K. (1981). Factors in the natural language of personality: Re-analysis, comparison, and interpretation of six major studies. *Multivariate Behavioral Research, 16,* 149-170.

Dishman, R. K. (1978). Aerobic power, estimation of physical ability, and attraction to physical activity. *Research Quarterly, 49,* 285-292.

Dishman, R. K. (1982). Compliance/adherence in health-related exercise. *Health Psychology, 1,* 237-267.

Dishman, R. K. (1984). Motivation and exercise adherence. In J. M. Silva, III & R. S. Weinberg (Eds.), *Psychological foundations of sport.* Champaign, IL: Human Kinetics.

Dishman, R. K. (1985). Medical psychology in exercise and sport. *Medical Clinics of North America, 69,* 123-143.

Dishman, R. K., & Ickes, W. (1981). Self-motivation and adherence to therapeutic exercise. *Journal of Behavioral Medicine, 4,* 421-438.

Dishman, R. K., Ickes, W., & Morgan, W. P. (1980). Self-motivation and adherence to habitual physical exercise. *Journal of Applied Social Psychology, 10,* 115-132.

Dishman, R. K., Sallis, J. F., & Orenstein, D. R. (1985). The determinants of physical activity and exercise. *Public Health Reports, 100,* 158-171.

Doan, R. E., & Scherman, A. (1987). The therapeutic effect of physical fitness on measures of personality: A literature review. *Journal of Counseling and Development, 66,* 28-36.

Dodson, L. C., & Mullens, W. R. (1969). Some effects of jogging on psychiatric hospital patients. *American Correctional Therapy Journal, 23,* 130-134.

Doyne, E. J., Ossip-Klein, D. J., Bowman, E. D., Osborn, K. M., McDougall-Wilson, I. B., & Neimeyer, R. A. (1987). Running versus weight lifting in the treatment of depression. *Journal of Consulting and Clinical Psychology, 55,* 748-754.

Dreger, R. M. (1978). The State-Trait Anxiety Inventory. In O. K. Buros (Ed.), *The eighth mental measurements yearbook* (pp. 1094-1095). Highland Park, NJ: Gryphon Press.

Dulberg, H. N., & Bennett, F. W. (1980). Psychological changes in early adolescent males induced by systematic exercise. *American Correctional Therapy Journal, 34,* 142-146.

Eichman, W. J. (1978). Profile of Mood States. In O. K. Buros (Ed.), *The eighth mental measurements yearbook* (pp. 1016-1018). Highland Park, NJ: Gryphon Press.

Eichner, E. R. (1983). Exercise and heart disease: Epidemiology of the "exercise hypothesis." *American Journal of Medicine, 75,* 1008-1023.

Eickhoff, J., Thorland, W., & Ansorge, C. (1983). Selected physiological and psychological effects of aerobic dancing among young adult women. *Journal of Sports Medicine and Physical Fitness, 23,* 273-280.

El-Naggar, A. M. (1986). Physical training effect on relationship of physical, mental, and emotional fitness in
adult men. *Journal of Human Ergology, 15,* 79-84.
Emory, J. F. (1980). *An analysis of the correlates of body
image of the members of the Adult Health and Development Program at the University of Maryland.* Unpub-
lished master's thesis, University of Maryland, College
Park, MD.
Epstein, J. H. (1985). Piers-Harris Self-Concept Scale. In
J. V. Mitchell, Jr. (Ed.), *The ninth mental measurements
yearbook* (pp. 1167-1169). Lincoln, NE: University of
Nebraska Press.
Eysenck, H. J. (1978). A exercise in mega-silliness. *Amer-
ican Psychologist, 33,* 517.
Eysenck, H. J., & Eysenck, S. (1963). *Manual for the Ey-
senck Personality Inventory.* San Diego: Educational and
Industrial Testing Service.
Eysenck, H. J., Nias, D. K. B., & Cox, D. N. (1982). Sport
and personality. *Advances in Behavior Research and
Therapy, 4,* 1-55.
Fiske, D. W. (1983). The meta-analytic revolution in out-
come research. *Journal of Consulting and Clinical Psy-
chology, 51,* 65-70.
Fitts, W. H. (1965). *Manual for Tennessee Self Concept
Scale.* Los Angeles: Western Psychological Services.
Fixx, J. F. (1977). *The complete book of running.* New
York: Random House.
Fixx, J. F. (1980). *Jim Fixx's second book of running.* New
York: Random House.
Folkins, C. H. (1976). Effects of physical training on mood.
Journal of Clinical Psychology, 32, 385-388.
Folkins, C. H., Lynch, S., & Gardner, M. M. (1972). Psy-
chological fitness as a function of physical fitness. *Ar-
chives of Physical Medicine and Rehabilitation, 53,*
503-508.
Folkins, C. H., & Sime, W. E. (1981). Physical fitness
training and mental health. *American Psychologist, 36,*
373-389.
Fox, K. R., & Corbin, C. B. (1989). The Physical Self-
Perception Profile: Development and preliminary validation. *Journal of Sport and Exercise Psychology, 11,*
408-430.
Fox, K. R., Corbin, C. B., & Couldry, W. H. (1985). Female
physical estimation and attraction to physical activity.
Journal of Sport Psychology, 7, 125-136.
Frankel, A., & Murphy, J. (1974). Physical fitness and
personality in alcoholism. *Quarterly Journal of Studies
on Alcoholism, 35,* 1272-1278.
Franklin, B. A., & Rubenfire, M. (1980). Losing weight
through exercise. *Journal of the American Medical Association, 244,* 377-379.
Frazier, S. E., & Nagy, S. (1989). Mood state changes of
women as a function of regular aerobic exercise. *Perceptual and Motor Skills, 68,* 283-287.
Gary, V., & Guthrie, D. (1972). The effect of jogging on
physical fitness and self-concept in hospitalized alcoholics. *Quarterly Journal of Studies on Alcoholism, 33,*
1073-1078.

Gillick, M. R. (1984). Health promotion, jogging, and the pursuit of the moral life. *Journal of Health Politics, Policy and Law, 9,* 369-387.

Gillum, R. F., Folsom, A. R., & Blackburn, H. (1984). Decline in coronary heart disease mortality: Old questions and new facts. *The American Journal of Medicine, 76,* 1055-1065.

Glass, G. V. (1976). Primary, secondary, and meta-analysis of research. *Educational Researcher, 5,* 3-8.

Glass, G. V., McGaw, B., & Smith, M. L. (1981). *Meta-analysis in social research.* Beverly Hills, CA: Sage.

Goff, D., and Dimsdale, J. E. (1985). The psychologic effects of exercise. *Journal of Cardiopulmonary Rehabilitation, 5,* 234-240.

Goldberg, A. P., Hagberg, J., Delmez, J. A., Carney, R. M., McKevitt, P. M., Ehsani, A. A., & Harter, H. R. (1980). The metabolic and psychological effects of exercise training in hemodialysis patients. *American Journal of Clinical Nutrition, 33,* 1620-1628.

Goldwater, B. C., & Collis, M. L. (1985). Psychologic effects of cardiovascular conditioning: A controlled experiment. *Psychosomatic Medicine, 47,* 174-181.

Gondola, J. C., & Tuckman, B. W. (1982). Psychological mood state in "average" marathon runners. *Perceptual and Motor Skills, 55,* 1295-1300.

Gondola, J. C., & Tuckman, B. W. (1983). Extent of training and mood enhancement in women runners. *Perceptual and Motor Skills, 57,* 333-334.

Goodstein, L. D. (1972a). The Depression Adjective Check Lists. In O. K. Buros (Ed.), *The seventh mental measurements yearbook* (pp. 132-133). Highland Park, NJ: Gryphon Press.

Goodstein, L. D. (1972b). The Self-Rating Depression Scale. In O. K. Buros (Ed.), *The seventh mental measurements yearbook* (pp. 320-321). Highland Park, NJ: Gryphon Press.

Gough, H. G. (1955). *Reference handbook for the Gough Adjective Check-List.* Berkeley, CA: University of California Institute for Personality Assessment and Research.

Gough, H. G. (1960). The Adjective Check List as a personality assessment research technique. *Psychological Reports, 6,* 107-122.

Green, B. F., & Hall, J. A. (1984). Quantitative methods for literature reviews. *Annual Review of Psychology, 35,* 37-53.

Greist, J. H., Klein, M. H., Eischens, R. R., Faris, J., Gurman, A. S., & Morgan, W. P. (1981). Running through your mind. In M. H. Sacks & M. L. Sachs (Eds.), *Psychology of running* (pp. 5-31). Champaign, IL: Human Kinetics Publishers.

Griffin, S. J., & Trinder, J. (1978). Physical fitness, exercise, and human sleep. *Psychophysiology, 15,* 447-450.

Hammer, W. M., & Wilmore, J. H. (1973). An exploratory investigation in personality measures and physiological alterations during a 10-week jogging program. *Journal of Sports Medicine. 13,* 238-247.

Hammett, V. B. O. (1967). Psychological changes with physical fitness training. *Canadian Medical Association Journal, 96,* 764-769.

Hannaford, C. P., Harrell, E. H., & Cox, K. (1988). Psychophysiological effects of a running program on depression and anxiety in a psychiatric population. *Psychological Record, 38,* 37-48.

Hanson, J. S., & Nedde, W. H. (1974). Long-term physical training effect in sedentary females. *Journal of Applied Physiology, 37,* 112-116.

Harsh, C. M. (1953). The 16PF Questionnaire. In O. K. Buros (Ed.), *The fourth mental measurements yearbook* (pp. 147-148). Highland Park, NJ: Gryphon Press.

Hartung, G. H., & Farge, E. J. (1979). Personality and physiological traits in middle-aged runners and joggers. *Journal of Gerontology, 32,* 541-548.

Hartung, G. H., Foreyt, J. P., Mitchell, R. E., Vlasek, I., & Gotto, A. M., Jr. (1980). Relation of diet to high-density lipoprotein cholesterol in middle-aged marathon runners, joggers, and inactive men. *New England Journal of Medicine, 302,* 357-361.

Haskell, W. L. (1984). Overview: Health benefits of exercise. In J. D. Matarazzo, S. M. Weiss, J. A. Herd, N. E. Miller, & S. M. Weiss (Eds.), *Behavioral health: A handbook of health enhancement and disease prevention* (pp. 409-423). New York: John Wiley.

Hathaway, S. R., & McKinley, J. C. (1943). *Minnesota Multiphasic Personality Inventory.* New York: The Psychological Corporation.

Hayden, R. M., & Allen, G. J. (1984). Relationship between aerobic exercise, anxiety, and depression: Convergent validation by knowledgeable informants. *Journal of Sports Medicine and Physical Fitness, 24,* 69-74.

Hedges, L. V. (1981). Distribution theory for Glass's estimator of effect size and related estimators. *Journal of Educational Statistics, 6,* 107-128.

Hedges, L. V. (1982). Estimation of effect size from a series of independent experiments. *Psychological Bulletin, 92,* 490-499.

Hedges, L. V., & Olkin, I. (1985). *Statistical methods for meta-analysis.* Orlando, FL: Academic Press.

Heilbrun, A. B. (1958). Relationships between the Adjective Check-List, Personal Preference Schedule, and desirability factors under varying defensiveness conditions. *Journal of Clinical Psychology, 14,* 283-287.

Heilbrun, A. B. (1959). Validation of a need scaling technique for the Adjective Check List. *Journal of Consulting Psychology, 23,* 347-351.

Hilyer, J. C., Jr., & Mitchell, W. (1979). Effect of systematic physical fitness training combined with counseling on the self-concept of college students. *Journal of Counseling Psychology, 26,* 427-436.

Hogan, J. (1989). Personality correlates of physical fitness. *Journal of Personality and Social Psychology, 56,* 284-288.

Howell, M. L., & Alderman, R. B. (1967). Psychological determinants of fitness. *Canadian Medical Association Journal, 96,* 721-728.

Hughes, J. R. (1984). Psychological effects of habitual aerobic exercise: A critical review. *Preventive Medicine,
13*, 66-78.

Ismail, A. H., & Young, R. J. (1973). The effect of chronic
exercise on the personality of middle-aged men by uni-
variate and multivariate approaches. *Journal of Human
Ergology, 2*, 47-57.

Ismail, A. H., & Young, R. J. (1977). Effect of chronic
exercise on the personality of adults. *Annals of the New
York Academy of Science, 301*, 958-969.

Jackson, G. B. (1980). Methods for integrative reviews.
Review of Educational Research, 50, 438-460.

Jasnoski, M. L., & Holmes, D. S. (1981). Influence of initial
aerobic fitness, aerobic training and changes in aerobic
fitness on personality functioning. *Journal of Psychosomatic Research, 25*, 553-556.

Jette, M. (1975). Habitual exercisers: A blood serum and
personality profile. *Journal of Sports Medicine, 3*, 12-17.

Joesting, J., & Clance, P. R. (1979). Comparison of runners
and nonrunners on the body-cathexis and self-cathexis
scales. *Perceptual and Motor Skills, 48*, 1046.

Johnson, A., Collins, P., Higgins, I., Harrington, D., Con-
nolly, J., Dolphin, C., McCreery, M., Brady, L., &
O'Brien, M. (1985). Psychological, nutritional and physical status of olympic road cyclists. *British Journal of
Sports Medicine, 19*, 11-14.

Jones, L. Y. (1980). *Great expectations: America and the
baby boom generation.* New York: Ballantine.

Jones, R. D., & Weinhouse, S. (1979). Running as self
therapy. *Journal of Sports Medicine and Physical Fitness, 19*, 397-404.

Jorgenson, G., Jansen, F., & Samuelson, C. (1968). *Inter-
personal relationships: Factors in job placement.* Salt
Lake City, UT: University of Utah, Department of Educational Psychology.

Katkin, E. S. (1978). The State-Trait Anxiety Inventory. In
O. K. Buros (Ed.), *The eighth mental measurements
yearbook* (pp. 1095-1096). Highland Park, NJ: Gryphon
Press.

Kavanagh, T., Shephard, R. J., Tuck, J. A., & Qureshi, S.
(1977). Depression following myocardial infarction: The
effects of distance running. *Annals of the New York
Academy of Science, 301*, 1029-1038.

Kelly, E. L. (1972). The Multiple Affect Adjective Check
List. In O. K. Buros (Ed.) *The seventh mental meas-
urements yearbook* (pp. 271-272). Highland Park, NJ:
Gryphon Press.

Klein, M. H., Greist, J. H., Gurman, A. S., Neimeyer, R.
A., Lesser, D. P., Bushnell, N. J., & Smith, R. E. (1985).
A comparative outcome study of group psychotherapy
vs. exercise treatments for depression. *International
Journal of Mental Health, 13*, 148-177.

Kline, P. (1978). The Eysenck Personality Questionnaire. In
O. K. Buros (Ed.), *The eighth mental measurements
yearbook* (pp. 809-810). Highland Park, NJ: Gryphon
Press.

Kowal, D. M., Patton, J. F., & Vogel, J. A. (1978). Psychological states and aerobic fitness of male and female

recruits before and after basic training. *Aviation, Space, and Environmental Medicine, 49,* 603-606.

Lambert, C. A., Netherton, D. R., Finison, L. J., Hyde, J. N., & Spaight, S. J. (1982). Risk factors and life style: A statewide health-interview survey. *New England Journal of Medicine, 306,* 1048-1051.

Landman, J. T., & Dawes, R. M. (1982). Psychotherapy outcome: Smith and Glass' conclusions stand up under scrutiny. *American Psychologist, 37,* 504-516.

Layman, E. McC. (1974). Psychological effects of physical activity. *Exercise and Sport Science Reviews. 2,* 33-70.

Ledwidge, B. (1980). Run for your mind: Aerobic exercise as a means of alleviating anxiety and depression. *Canadian Journal of Behavioral Science, 12,* 126-140.

Leonardson, G. R., & Gargiulo, R. M. (1978). Self-perception and physical fitness. *Perceptual and Motor Skills, 46,* 338.

Leste, A., & Rust, J. (1984). Effects of dance on anxiety. *Perceptual and Motor Skills, 58,* 767-772.

Levy, R. I., & Moskowitz, J. (1982). Cardiovascular research: Decades of progress, a decade of promise. *Science, 217,* 121-129.

Light, R. J., & Smith, P. V. (1971). Accumulating evidence: Procedures for resolving contradictions among different research studies. *Harvard Educational Review, 41,* 429-471.

Lobstein, D. D., Mosbacher, B. J., & Ismail, A. H. (1983). Depression as a powerful discriminator between physically active and sedentary middle-aged men. *Journal of Psychosomatic Research, 27,* 69-76.

Loehlin, J. C. (1987). *Latent variable models: An introduction to factor, path, and structural analysis.* Hillsdale, NJ: Lawrence Erlbaum.

Long, B. C., & Haney, C. J. (1988). Coping strategies for working women: Aerobic exercise and relaxation interventions. *Behavior Therapy, 19,* 75-83.

Lubin, A. (1953). The 16PF Questionnaire. In O. K. Buros (Ed.), *The fourth mental measurements yearbook* (p. 148). Highland Park, NJ: Gryphon Press.

Lubin, B. (1965). Adjective checklists for measurement of depression. *Archives of General Psychiatry, 12,* 57-62.

Lubin, B. (1981). *Depression Adjective Check Lists.* San Diego: Educational and Industrial Testing Service.

Lunde, A. S. (1981). Health in the United States. *Annals of the American Academy of Political and Social Science. 453,* 28-69.

Lykken, D. T. (1968). Statistical significance in psychological research. *Psychological Bulletin, 70,* 151-159.

MacMahon, J. R., & Gross, R. T. (1987). Physical and psychological effects of aerobic exercise in boys with learning disabilities. *Journal of Developmental and Behavioral Pediatrics, 8,* 274-277.

Madden, D. J., Blumenthal, J. A., Allen, P. A., & Emery, C. F. (1989). Improving aerobic capacity in healthy older adults does not necessarily lead to improved cognitive performance. *Psychology and Aging, 4,* 307-320.

Maloney, J. P., Cheney, R., Spring, W., & Kanusky, J. (1986). The physiologic and psychological effects of a

5-week and a 16-week physical fitness program. *Military Medicine, 151,* 426-433.

Mansfield, R. S., & Busse, T. V. (1977). Meta-analysis of research: A rejoinder to Glass. *Educational Researcher, 6,* 3.

Marsh, H. W., & Peart, N. D. (1988). Competitive and co-operative physical fitness training programs for girls: Effects on physical fitness and multidimensional self-concepts. *Journal of Sport and Exercise Psychology, 10,* 390-407.

Marshall, E. (1980). Psychotherapy works, but for whom? *Science, 207,* 506-508.

Martin, J. E., & Dubbert, P. M. (1982). Exercise applications and promotion in behavioral medicine: Current status and future directions. *Journal of Consulting and Clinical Psychology, 50,* 1004-1017.

Matarazzo, J. D. (1982). Behavioral health's challenge to academic, scientific, and professional psychology. *American Psychologist, 37,* 1-14.

Matarazzo, J. D. (1984). Behavioral health: A 1990 challenge for the health sciences professions. In J. D. Matarazzo, S. M. Weiss, J. A. Herd, N. E. Miller, & S. M. Weiss (Eds.), *Behavioral health: A handbook of health enhancement and disease prevention* (pp. 3-40). New York: John Wiley.

McCann, I. L., & Holmes, D. S. (1984). Influence of aerobic exercise on depression. *Journal of Personality and Social Psychology, 46,* 1142-1147.

McDonald, D. G., Beckett, M. B., & Hodgdon, J. A. (1991). Psychological predictors of physical performance and fitness in U.S. Navy personnel. *Military Psychology, 3,* 73-87.

McDonald, D. G., & Manley, C. M. (1991). *A general model of the role of mediators in the effects of exercise and fitness on self-esteem.* Unpublished manuscript.

McDonald, D. G., Norton, J. P., & Hodgdon, J. A. (1990). Training success in U.S. Navy Special Forces. *Aviation, Space, and Environmental Medicine, 61,* 548-554.

McGlynn, G. H., Franklin, B., Lauro, G., & McGlynn, I. K. (1983). The effect of aerobic conditioning and induced stress on state-trait anxiety, blood pressure, and muscle tension. *Journal of Sports Medicine, 23,* 341-351.

McGowan, R. W., Jarman, B. O., & Pedersen, D. M. (1974). Effects of a competitive endurance training program on self-concept and peer approval. *Journal of Psychology, 86,* 57-60.

McNair, D. M. (1972). The Depression Adjective Check Lists. In O. K. Buros (Ed.), *The seventh mental measurements yearbook* (pp. 133-134). Highland Park, NJ: Gryphon Press.

McNair, D. M., Lorr, M., & Droppleman, L. F. (1971). *Manual for the Profile of Mood States.* San Diego: Educational and Industrial Testing Service.

Megargee, E. I. (1972). The Multiple Affect Adjective Check List. In O. K. Buros (Ed.), *The seventh mental measurements yearbook* (pp. 272-274). Highland Park, NJ: Gryphon Press.

Mellion, M. B. (1985). Exercise therapy for anxiety and depression: 1. Does the evidence justify its recommendation? *Postgraduate Medicine, 77,* 59-62, 66.

Mihevic, P. M. (1982). Anxiety, depression, and exercise. *Quest, 33,* 140-153.

Mikel, K. V. (1983). Extraversion in adult runners. *Perceptual and Motor Skills, 57,* 143-146.

Morgan, W. P. (1985). Affective beneficence of vigorous physical activity. *Medicine and Science in Sports and Exercise, 17,* 94-100.

Morgan, W. P., & Costill, D. L. (1972). Psychological characteristics of the marathon runner. *Journal of Sports Medicine, 12,* 42-46.

Morgan, W. P., & Goldston, S. E. (Eds.). (1987). *Exercise and mental health* New York: Hemisphere.

Morgan, W. P., O'Connor, P. J., Ellickson, K. A., & Bradley, P. W. (1988). Personality structure, mood states, and performance in elite male distance runners. *International Journal of Sport Psychology, 19,* 247-263.

Morgan, W. P., O'Connor, P. J., Sparling, P. B., & Pate, R. R. (1987). Psychological characterization of the elite female distance runner. *International Journal of Sports Medicine, 8,* 124-131.

Morgan, W. P., & Pollock, M. L. (1977). Psychologic characterization of the elite distance runner. *Annals of the New York Academy of Sciences, 301,* 382-403.

Morgan, W. P., Roberts, J. A., Brand, F. R., & Feinerman, A. D. (1970). Psychological effect of chronic physical activity. *Medicine and Science in Sports, 2,* 213-217.

Morris, A. F., & Husman, B. F. (1978). Life quality changes following an endurance conditioning program. *American Correctional Therapy Journal, 32,* 3-6.

Moses, J., Steptoe, A., Mathews, A., & Edwards, S. (1989). The effects of exercise training on mental well-being in the normal population: A controlled trial. *Journal of Psychosomatic Research, 33,* 47-61.

Nagy, S., & Frazier, S. E. (1988). The impact of exercise on locus of control, self-esteem and mood states. *Journal of Social Behavior and Personality, 3,* 263-268.

Naughton, J., Bruhn, J. G., & Lategola, M. T. (1968). Effects of physical training on physiologic and behavioral characteristics of cardiac patients. *Archives of Physical Medicine and Rehabilitation, 49,* 131-137.

Nelson, L. R., & Furst, M. L. (1972). An objective study of the effects of expectation on competitive performance. *Journal of Psychology, 81,* 69-72.

Netz, Y., Tenenbaum, G., & Sagiv, M. (1988). Pattern of psychological fitness as related to pattern of physical fitness among older adults. *Perceptual and Motor Skills, 67,* 647-655.

Noakes, T. D., Opie, L. H., Rose, A. G., & Kleynhans, P. H. T. (1979). Autopsy-proved coronary atherosclerosis in marathon runners. *New England Journal of Medicine, 301,* 86-89.

Noller, P., Law, H., & Comrey, A. L. (1987). Cattell, Comrey, and Eysenck personality factors compared: More evidence for the five robust factors? *Journal of Personality and Social Psychology, 53,* 775-782.

Nouri, S., & Beer, J. (1989). Relations of moderate physical exercise to scores on hostility, aggression, and trait-anxiety. *Perceptual and Motor Skills, 68*, 1191-1194.

Osgood, C. E., Suci, G. J., & Tannenbaum, P. H. (1957). *The measurement of meaning.* Urbana, IL: University of Illinois Press.

Paffenbarger, R. S., Wing, A. L., Hyde, R. T., & Jung, D. L. (1983). Physical activity and incidence of hypertension in college alumni. *American Journal of Epidemiology, 117*, 245-257.

Parent, C. J., & Whall, A. L. (1984). Are physical activity, self-esteem, & depression related? *Journal of Gerontological Nursing, 10*, 8-11.

Pauker, J. D. (1985). The SCL-90. In J. V. Mitchell, Jr. (Ed.), *The ninth mental measurements yearbook* (pp. 1325-1326). Lincoln, NE: University of Nebraska Press.

Pauly, J. T., Palmer, J. A., Wright, C. C., & Pfeiffer, G. J. (1982). The effect of a 14-week employee fitness program on selected physiological and psychological parameters. *Journal of Occupational Medicine, 24*, 457-463.

Paxton, S. J., Trinder, J., & Montgomery, I. (1983). Does aerobic fitness affect sleep? *Psychophysiology, 20*, 320-324.

Paxton, S. J., Trinder, J., Shapiro, C. M., Adam, K., Oswald, I., & Graf, K. J. (1984). Effect of physical fitness and body composition on sleep and sleep-related hormone concentrations. *Sleep, 7*, 39-346.

Payne, R. W. (1985). The SCL-90. In J. V. Mitchell, Jr. (Ed.), *The ninth mental measurements yearbook* (pp. 1326-1329). Lincoln, NE: University of Nebraska Press.

Percy, L. E., Dziuban, C. D., & Martin, J. B. (1981). Analysis of effects of distance running on self-concepts of elementary students. *Perceptual and Motor Skills, 52*, 42.

Perri, S., II, & Templer, D. I. (1984-85). The effects of an aerobic exercise program on psychological variables in older adults. *International Journal of Aging and Human Development, 20*, 167-172.

Pflaum, J. H. (1973). *Development of a life quality inventory.* Unpublished doctoral dissertation, University of Maryland, College Park, MD.

Piers, E. V., & Harris, D. B. (1984). *Manual for Children's Self-concept Scale* (rev. ed.). Los Angeles: Western Psychological Services.

Plummer, O. K., & Koh, Y. O. (1987). Effect of "aerobics" on self-concepts of college women. *Perceptual and Motor Skills, 65*, 271-275.

Radloff, L. S. (1977). The CES-D scale: A self-report depression scale for research in the general population. *Applied Psychological Measurement, 1*, 385-401.

Rape, R. N. (1987). Running and depression. *Perceptual and Motor Skills, 64*, 1303-1310.

Renfrow, N. E., & Bolton, B. (1979). Personality characteristics associated with aerobic exercise in adult males. *Journal of Personality Assessment, 43*, 261-266.

Riddick, C. C., & Freitag, R. S. (1984). The impact of an aerobic fitness program on the body image of older women. *Activities, Adaptation & Aging, 6*, 59-70.

Rorer, L. G. (1972). The Adjective Check List. In O. K. Buros (Ed.), *The seventh mental measurements yearbook* (pp. 74-77). Highland Park, NJ: Gryphon Press.

Rosenberg, M. (1963). The association between self-esteem and anxiety. *Journal of Psychiatric Research, 1,* 35-152.

Rosenthal, R. (1979). The "file drawer problem" and tolerance for null results. *Psychological Bulletin, 86,* 638-641.

Rosenthal, R. (1984). *Meta-analytic procedures for social research.* Beverly Hills, CA: Sage.

Rosenthal, R., & Rubin, D. B. (1986). Meta-analytic procedures for combining studies with multiple effect sizes. *Psychological Bulletin, 99,* 400-406.

Rudy, E. B., & Estok, P. J. (1983). Intensity of jogging: Its relationship to selected physical and psychosocial variables in women. *Western Journal of Nursing Research, 5,* 325-336.

Sachs, M. L., & Buffone, G. W. (Eds.). (1984). *Running as therapy: An integrated approach.* Lincoln, NE: University of Nebraska Press.

Sachs, M. L., & Buffone, G. W. (Eds.). (1985). *Bibliography: Psychological considerations in exercise, including exercise as psychotherapy, exercise addiction, and the psychology of running.* Unpublished manuscript.

Sacks, M. H., & Sachs, M. L. (Eds.). (1981). *Psychology of running.* Champaign, IL: Human Kinetics.

Safrit, M. J., Wood, T. M., & Dishman, R. K. (1985). The factorial validity of the Physical Estimation and Attraction Scales for adults. *Journal of Sport Psychology, 7,* 166-190.

Scheuer, J., & Tipton, C. M. (1977). Cardiovascular adaptations to physical training. *Annual Review of Physiology, 39,* , 221-251.

Secord, P. F., & Jourard, S. M. (1953). The appraisal of body-cathexis: Body-cathexis and the self. *Journal of Consulting Psychology, 17,* 343-347.

Shapiro, D. A., & Shapiro, D. (1982). Meta-analysis of comparative outcome studies: A replication and refinement. *Psychological Bulletin, 92,* 581-604.

Sharp, M. W., & Reilley, R. R. (1975). The relationship of aerobic physical fitness to selected personality traits. *Journal of Clinical Psychology, 31,* 428-430.

Sheehan, G. A. (1975). *Dr. Sheehan on running.* Mountain View, CA: World.

Shephard, R. J. (1985). Factors influencing the exercise behaviour of patients. *Sports Medicine, 2,* 348-366.

Shephard, R. J., & Cox, M. (1980). Some characteristics of participants in an industrial fitness programme. *Canadian Journal of Applied Sports Science, 5,* 9-76.

Sherrill, C., Holguin, O., & Caywood, A. J. (1989). Fitness, attitude toward physical education, and self-concept of elementary school children. *Perceptual and Motor Skills, 69,* 411-414.

Short, M. A., DiCarlo, S., Steffee, W. P., & Pavlou, K. (1984). Effects of physical conditioning on self-concept of adult obese males. *Physical Therapy, 64,* 194-198.

Silva, J. M., & Shultz, B. B. (1984). Research in the psychology and therapeutics of running: A methodological and interpretive review. In M. L. Sachs & G. W. Buffone

(Eds.), *Running as therapy: An integrated approach* (pp. 304-320). Lincoln, NE: University of Nebraska Press.

Sime, W. E. (1984). Psychological benefits of exercise training in the healthy individual. In J. D. Matarazzo, S. M. Weiss, J. A. Herd, N. E. Miller, & S. M. Weiss (Eds.), *Behavioral health: A handbook of health enhancement and disease prevention* (pp. 488-508). New York: John Wiley.

Simons, C. W., & Birkimer, J. C. (1988). An exploration of factors predicting the effects of aerobic conditioning on mood state. *Journal of Psychosomatic Research, 32,* 63-75.

Sinyor, D., Schwartz, S. G., Peronnet, F., Brisson, G., & Seraganian, P. (1983). Aerobic fitness level and reactivity to psychosocial stress: Physiological, biochemical, and subjective measures. *Psychosomatic Medicine, 45,* 205-217.

Siscovick, D. S., LaPorte, R. E., & Newman, J. M. (1985). The disease-specific benefits and risks of physical activity and exercise. *Public Health Reports, 100,* 180-188.

Smith, D. M., Khairi, M. R. A., Norton, J., & Johnston, C. C., Jr. (1976). Age and activity effects on rate of bone mineral loss. *Journal of Clinical Investigation, 58,* 716-721.

Smith, E. L., Reddan, W., & Smith, P. E. (1981). Physical activity and calcium modalities for bone mineral increase in aged women. *Medicine and Science in Sports and Exercise, 13,* 60-64.

Smith, M. L. (1980). Sex bias in counseling and psychotherapy. *Psychological Bulletin, 87,* 392-407.

Smith, M. L., & Glass, G. V. (1977). Meta-analysis of psychotherapy outcome studies. *American Psychologist, 32,* 752-760.

Smith, M. L., Glass, G. V., & Miller, T. I. (1980). *The Benefits of psychotherapy.* Baltimore: Johns Hopkins University Press.

Sonstroem, R. J. (1974). Attitude testing examining certain psychological correlates of physical activity. *Research Quarterly, 45,* 93-103.

Sonstroem, R. J. (1978). Physical estimation and attraction scales: Rationale and research. *Medicine and Science in Sports, 10,* 97-102.

Sonstroem, R. J. (1984). Exercise and self-esteem. *Exercise and Sport Science Reviews, 12,* 123-155.

Sonstroem, R. J., & Morgan, W. P. (1989). Exercise and self-esteem: Rationale and model. *Medicine and Science in Sports and Exercise, 21,* 329-337.

Spielberger, C. D. (1983). *Manual for the State-Trait Anxiety Inventory (Form Y, Self-Evaluation Questionnaire).* Palo Alto, CA: Consulting Psychologists Press.

Spielberger, C. D., Gorsuch, R. L., & Lushene, R. (1970). *Manual for the State-Trait Anxiety Inventory (Self-Evaluation Questionnaire).* Palo Alto, CA: Consulting Psycholgists Press.

Stamler, J. (1973). Epidemiology of coronary heart disease. *Medical Clinics of North America, 57,* 5-46.

Stamler, J. (1985). The marked decline in coronary heart disease mortality rates in the United States, 1968-1981;

summary of findings and possible explanations. *Cardiology, 72,* 11-22.

Stanley, J. C. (1973). Designing psychological experiments. In B. Wolman (Ed.), *Handbook of general psychology* (pp. 90-106). Englewood Cliffs, NJ: Prentice-Hall.

Steptoe, A., Edwards. S., Moses, J., & Mathews, A. (1989). The effects of exercise training on mood and perceived coping ability in anxious adults from the general population. *Journal of Psychosomatic Research, 33,* 537-547.

Stern, M. J., & Cleary, P. (1981). National exercise and heart disease project: Psychosocial changes observed during a low-level exercise program. *Archives of Internal Medicine, 141,* 1463-1467.

Stricker, L: J. (1978). The Eysenck Personality Questionnaire. In O. K. Buros (Ed.), *The eighth mental measurements yearbook,* (pp. 810-814). Highland Park, NJ: Gryphon Press.

Suinn, R. M. (1972). The Tennessee Self Concept Scale. In O. K. Buros (Ed.), *The seventh mental measurements yearbook* (pp. 367-369). Highland Park, NJ: Gryphon Press.

Suominen-Troyer, S., Davis, K. J., Ismail, A. H., & Salvendy, G. (1986). Impact of physical fitness on strategy development in decision-making tasks. *Perceptual and Motor Skills, 62,* 71-77.

Taylor, C. B., Sallis, J. F., & Needle, R. (1985). The relation of physical activity and exercise to mental health. *Public Health Reports, 100,* 195-202.

Taylor, J. A. (1951). The relationship of anxiety to the conditioned eyelid response. *Journal of Experimental Psychology, 41,* 81-92.

Taylor, J. A. (1953). A personality scale of manifest anxiety. *Journal of Abnormal and Social Psychology, 48,* 285-290.

Teeter, P. A. (1985). The Adjective Check List. In J. V. Mitchell, Jr. (Ed.), *The ninth mental measurements yearbook* (pp. 50-52). Lincoln, NE: University of Nebraska Press.

Tellegen, A. (1978). The Eysenck Personality Inventory. In O. K. Buros (Ed.), *The eighth mental measurements yearbook,* (pp. 802-804). Highland Park, NJ: Gryphon Press.

Thom, T. J., & Kannel, W. B. (1981). Downward trend in cardiovascular mortality. *Annual Review of Medicine, 32,* 427-434.

Tillman, K. (1965). Relationship between physical fitness and selected personality traits. *Research Quarterly, 36,* 483-489.

Tomporowski, P. D., & Ellis, N. R. (1986). Effects of exercise on cognitive processes: A review. *Psychological Bulletin. 99,* 338-346.

Trinder, J., Paxton, S. J., Montgomery, I., & Fraser, G. (1985). Endurance as opposed to power training: Their effect on sleep. *Psychophysiology, 22,* 668-673.

Valliant, P. M., Bennie, F. A. B., & Valiant, J. J. (1981). Do marathoners differ from joggers in personality profile: A sports psychology approach. *Journal of Sports Medicine and Physical Fitness, 21,* 62-67.

Vance, F. L. (1972). The Adjective Check List. In O. K. Buros (Ed.), *The seventh mental measurements yearbook* (pp. 77-78). Highland Park, NJ: Gryphon Press.

Vanfraechem, J. H. P., & Vanfraechem-Raway, R. (1978). The influence of training upon physiological and psychological parameters in young athletes. *Journal of Sports Medicine and Physical Fitness, 18,* 175-182.

Walker, J. M., Floyd, T. C., Fein, G., Cavness, C., Lualhati, R., & Feinberg, I. (1978). Effects of exercise on sleep. *Journal of Applied Physiology, 44,* 945-951.

Walsh, J. A. (1978). The 16PF Questionnaire. In O. K. Buros (Ed.), *The eighth mental measurements yearbook* (pp. 1081-1083). Highland Park, NJ: Gryphon Press.

Weckowicz, T. E. (1978). The Profile of Mood States. In O. K. Buros (Ed.), *The eighth mental measurements yearbook* (pp. 1018-1019). Highland Park, NJ: Gryphon Press.

Weinstein, W. S., & Meyers, A. W. (1983). Running as treatment for depression: Is it worth it? *Journal of Sport Psychology, 5,* 288-301.

Wilfley, D., & Kunce, J. (1986). Differential physical and psychological effects of exercise. *Journal of Counseling Psychology, 33,* 337-342.

Williams, J. M., & Getty, D. (1986). Effect of levels of exercise on psychological mood states, physical fitness, and plasma beta-endorphin. *Perceptual and Motor Skills, 63,* 1099-1105.

Williams, R. S., & Wallace, A. G. (Eds.). (1989). *Biological effects of physical activity.* Champaign, IL: Human Kinetics Books.

Wittenborn, J. R. (1953). The 16PF Questionnaire. In O. K. Buros (Ed.), *The fourth mental measurements yearbook* (pp. 148-149). Highland Park, NJ: Gryphon Press.

World Health Organization. (1983). *Primary prevention of essential hypertension.* Geneva: Author.

Wortman, P. M. (1983). Evaluation research: A methodological perspective. *Annual Review of Psychology, 34,* 223-260.

Young, M. L. (1985). Estimation of fitness and physical ability, physical performance, and self-concept among adolescent females. *Journal of Sports Medicine, 25,* 144-150.

Young, R. J. (1979). The effect of regular exercise on cognitive functioning and personality. *British Journal of Sports Medicine, 13,* 110-117.

Young, R. J., & Ismail, A. H. (1976). Personality differences of adult men before and after a physical fitness program. *Research Quarterly, 47,* 513-519.

Zarske, J. A. (1985). The Adjective Check List. In J. V. Mitchell, Jr. (Ed.), *The ninth mental measurements yearbook* (pp. 52-53). Lincoln, NE: University of Nebraska Press.

Zloty, R. B., Burdick, J. A., & Adamson, J. D. (1973). Sleep of distance runners. *Activitas Nervosa Superior, 15,* 217-221.

Zuckerman, M. (1985). The 16PF Questionnaire. In J. V. Mitchell, Jr. (Ed.), *The ninth mental measurements yearbook* (pp. 1392-1394). Lincoln, NE: University of Nebraska Press.

Zuckerman, M., & Lubin, B. (1965). *Manual for the Multiple Affect Adjective Check List.* San Diego: Educational and Industrial Testing Service.

Zung, W. W. K. (1965). A self-rating depression scale. *Archives of General Psychiatry, 12,* 63-70.

Zung, W. W. K. (1969). A cross-cultural survey of symptoms in depression. *American Journal of Psychiatry, 126,* 116-121.

INDEX